s book is to be returned on or before the
last date stamped below

The Effective Management of Chronic Lymphocytic Leukaemia

The Effective Management of Chronic Lymphocytic Leukaemia

Edited by

Terry Hamblin DM FRCP FRCPath FMedSci
Professor of Immunohaematology & Chairman, UK CLL Forum
University of Southampton

Steve Johnson MB BS FRCP FRCPath
Consultant Haematologist, Taunton Hospital, Somerset
and Secretary, Haemato-oncology Task Force
of the British Society for Haematology Committee
for Standards in Haematology

Andrew Miles MSc MPhil PhD
Professor of Public Health Sciences
and Editor-in-Chief, Journal of Evaluation in Clinical Practice
Barts and The London,
Queen Mary's School of Medicine and Dentistry
University of London, UK

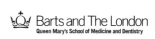

The Royal College
of
Radiologists

Association of
Cancer
Physicians

THE UK CLL FORUM

AESCULAPIUS MEDICAL PRESS
LONDON SAN FRANCISCO SYDNEY

Published by

Aesculapius Medical Press (London, San Francisco, Sydney)
PO Box LB48, Mount Pleasant Mail Centre, Farringdon Road, London EC1A 1LB, UK

© Aesculapius Medical Press 2004

First published 2004

British Library Cataloguing in Publication Data
A CIP catalogue record for this book is available from the British Library

ISBN 1 903044 44 8

While the advice and information in this book are believed to be true and accurate at the
time of going to press, neither the authors nor the publishers nor the sponsoring institutions
can accept any legal responsibility or liability for any errors or omissions that may be made.
In particular (but without limiting the generality of the preceding disclaimer) every effort
has been made to check drug usages; however, it is possible that errors have been missed.
Furthermore, dosage schedules are constantly being revised and new side effects recognised.
For these reasons, the reader is strongly urged to consult the drug companies' printed
instructions before administering any of the drugs recommended in this book.

Further copies of this volume are available from:

Claudio Melchiorri
Aesculapius Medical Press
PO Box LB48, Mount Pleasant Mail Centre, Farringdon Road, London EC1A 1LB, UK

Fax: 020 8525 8661
Email: claudio@keyadvances4.demon.co.uk
www.keyadvances.org.uk

Copy edited by The Clyvedon Press Ltd, Cardiff, UK

Typeset, printed and bound in Britain
Peter Powell Origination & Print Limited

Contents

Contributors

David J. Allsup BSc MBChB MRCP DipRCPath, Clinical Lecturer, Department of Haematology, University of Liverpool, UK

Bruno Cazin MD, Consultant Haematologist, University Hospital CHRU Huriez, Lille, France

Daniel Catovsky DSc FRCP FRCPath FMedSci, Professor Emeritus, The Institute of Cancer Research and Royal Marsden Hospital NHS Trust, London, UK

John C. Cawley MBChB MD PhD FRCP FRCPath FMedSci, Professor of Haematology/Honorary Consultant, Department of Haematology, University of Liverpool, UK

Martin J. S. Dyer MA DPhil FRCP FRCPath, Professor of Haemato-Oncology and Honorary Consultant Physician, MRC Toxicology Unit / Leicester University Hodgkin Building, Leicester, UK

Anne C. Gardiner BSc, Clinical Cytogeneticist, Department of Haematology, Royal Bournemouth Hospital, Bournemouth, UK

Terry J. Hamblin DM FRCP FRCPath FMedSci, Professor of Immunohaematology, University of Southampton & Chairman, UK CLL Forum

Richard S. Houlston MD PhD FRCPath FRCP, Reader in Molecular and Population Genetics, Institute of Cancer Research, Sutton, Surrey, UK

Stephen A. Johnson MBBS FRCP FRCPath, Consultant Haematologist, Taunton & Somerset Hospital, Taunton, UK & Secetary, Haemato-oncology Task Force of the BSH Committee for Standards in Haematology

Zoltan Matrai MD, Consultant Haematologist, Department of Haematology, University of Liverpool, UK

Estella Matutes MD PhD FRCPath, Reader and Consultant Haematologist, Royal Marsden Hospital and Institute of Cancer Research, London, UK

Donald W. Milligan MD FRCP FRCPath, Reader in Haematology & Consultant Haematologist, Birmingham Heartlands Hospital & Chairman, Haemato-oncology Task Force of the BSH Committee for Standards in Haematology

Paul Moss PhD FRCP FRCPath, Professor of Haematology, University of Birmingham, UK

David G. Oscier FRCP FRCPath, Consultant Haematologist, Department of Haematology, Royal Bournemouth Hospital, Bournemouth, UK

Andrew Pettitt MA MB BChir PhD MRCP MRCPath, Senior Lecturer/Honorary Consultant, Department of Haematology, University of Liverpool, UK

Gabrielle Sellick BSc PhD, Post-doctoral Research Fellow, Institute of Cancer Research, Sutton, Surrey, UK

Paul D. Sherrington MSc PhD, Clinical Scientist/Honorary Lecturer, Department of Haematology, University of Liverpool, UK

Mirko Zuzel MD, Reader in Haematology, Department of Haematology, University of Liverpool, UK

Preface

In Western countries, leukaemia affects about 1–2% of the population with B-cell chronic lymphocytic leukaemia (CLL), one of the most intruiging of the lymphoid neoplasms, representing the most common form of leukaemia, accounting for approximately 30% of all cases. Evidence from epidemiological studies strongly supports the notion that a subset of CLL involves inherited susceptibility and multiple reports of familial clustering indicate that first-degree relatives of individuals with CLL have a two to sevenfold excess risk of developing the disease. It is probable that, in addition to alleles conferring a significant genetic risk, part of the inherited susceptibility to the disease is mediated through numerous low-risk alleles. Importantly, the identification of the genes involved in familial forms of CLL should provide insights into the pathogenesis of CLL in general and it is for this reason that dense genome-wide linkage studies and highly empowered linkage studies should now become the subject of urgent research, as Sellick, Catovsky and Houlston emphasise within their elegantly written chapter which opens Part One of this volume.

Early cytogenetic studies in CLL performed in the 1960s and 1970s failed to detect clonal cytogenetic abnormalities, an inauspicious start to the investigation of genetic abnormalities in CLL that was the consequence of the low spontaneous mitotic rate in CLL and the use of the T-cell mitogen phytohaemaglutinin to obtain analysable metaphases. Following the discovery of the polyclonal B cell mitogens, the first cytogenetic abnormality in CLL (trisomy 12) was discovered, relatively recently, in 1980. Subsequent studies employed tetradecanoyl phorbol acetate (TPA) as a mitogen and demonstrated clonal cytogenetic abnormalities in approximately 50% of cases of CLL. The most frequent abnormalities are structural abnormalities of chromosome 13q14 and trisomy of chromosome 12, occurring in around 10–20% of cases, in contrast, therefore, to abnormalities in chromosomes 6q, 11q, 14q and 17p, which are each found in less than 5% of cases of CLL. It is to a particularly detailed discussion of these cytogenetic abnormalities in CLL and their analysis that Oscier and Gardiner turn in Chapter Two.

In Chapter Three, which completes Part One of the volume, Pettitt and his colleagues contribute an in-depth review of the natural history of CLL. As these authors show, the uniformity of morphology and immunophenotype of the malignant lymphocytes belies a truly remarkable variation in clinical behaviour and outcome, the biological basis of which has only just started to be unravelled. Their chapter details the events both before and after diagnosis (as the latter is a meaningless biological milestone in the asymptomatic patient whose disease is detected incidentally). Importantly, Pettitt and associates address several questions of central relevance to a proper understanding of the pathogenesis of CLL, including: 'How should CLL be defined, and how does it relate to small lymphocytic lymphoma

(SLL) and the recently described 'monoclonal lymphocytosis of undetermined significance (MLUS)?'; 'Who gets CLL in terms of age, sex and geography, and what can be deduced from this?'; 'What is the normal counterpart of the CLL cell, and should the disease be regarded as one or more than one entity on the basis of the cell of origin?'; 'What role do antigenic stimulation and the micro-environment play in the development and perpetuation of CLL, and does this have any implications for novel therapeutic approaches?'; 'Why is CLL associated with immune dysregulation?'; 'Why is there such a wide variation in organ involvement between individual patients, and is cell trafficking a potential target for therapeutic intervention?'; 'Why do the kinetics of disease progression, response to therapy and survival vary so widely between individual patients?' and 'What impact does treatment have on the natural history of CLL?'.

We have dedicated Part Two of the volume, through Chapters 4–7, to a detailed review of the evidence and opinion base for medical intervention in CLL. In the opening chapter of this Part, Matutes reviews current approaches to the diagnosis and classification of CLL. As she emphasises, the diagnosis of CLL needs to be based on a constellation of clinical and laboratory features and morphology and immunological markers are the two key initial tests that make it possible to establish the diagnosis of CLL in the majority of patients. She is clear that in a minority of cases with atypical morphology and/or immunophenotype, these tests should be complemented with others, e.g., fluorescence *in situ* hybridization (FISH) and/or histology to confirm the diagnosis of CLL and thus to rule out other B-cell lymphoproliferative disorders. According to the morphology, CLL can, as she shows, be classified into two groups: *typical* and *atypical*. In typical CLL, more than 90% of circulating lymphocytes are small, have a clumped nuclear chromatin and no visible or unconspicuous nucleoli; few prolymphocytoid cells may be seen, but these account for less than 10% of cells. Approximately, 15% of cases are atypical and these comprise CLL with greater that 10% prolymphocytes (CLL/PL) and CLL with more than 15% lymphoplasmacytoid and/or cleaved cells (mixed CLL according to the FAB).

Immunophenotype, as Matutes discusses, is a robust index for establishing the diagnosis of chronic lymphocytic leukaemia. Indeed, CLL cells have a distinct immunophenotypic profile: they express weak Ig in the surface, are CD5 and CD23 positive and FMC7 negative; CD22 and CD79b are weakly expressed or negative. While none of these markers are specific for CLL, they allow us, when compounded into a scoring system, to distinguish CLL from other B-cell leukaemias and lymphomas. Scores in CLL are 4 or 5 and rarely 3, while scores in the other diseases are, generally, under 3. Despite the fact that FMC7 recognises a particular epitope of CD20, its substitution in the scoring by CD20, decreases significantly its diagnostic power as most CLL cases weakly express CD20. Other markers such as CD38, ZAP-70, p53 have a prognostic impact but do not help in the diagnosis, as Matutes shows. In cases with atypical morphology and/or immunophenotype, FISH analysis investigating the presence of t(11;14), t(14;18) and trisomy 12 is essential, particularly when a diagnosis of mantle cell or follicular lymphoma is being considered. Bone marrow histology may be of additional use by demonstrating the presence of proliferating centres not seen in B-cell lymphomas. Beyond the diagnostic value of morphology and immunological markers, some of these investigations have prognostic significance and Matutes is clear that they should routinely and systematically be carried out in a diagnostic work-up of CLL.

In the chapter which follows, Hamblin reviews modern prognostic factors for CLL, their impact on the treatment of early disease and the place of 'watchful waiting' as part of the effective management of CLL. A meta-analysis of over 2000 early stage patients with CLL, randomised between early treatment and watchful waiting, showed no advantage for either approach and for several years it has therefore been considered good practice to delay treatment until progression in Binet stage A disease. However, recent advances in treatment and diagnosis have, as Hamblin discusses, challenged that conclusion. For example, it is, as he points out, well known that in some patients CLL is a very indolent condition with some patients surviving for decades without progression and dying of an irrelevant cause without ever requiring treatment for their disease. It is also recognised that the treatment of advanced stage CLL is never curative, except perhaps in a small minority of patients treated by stem cell allograft. The meta-analysis cited concerned all early stage patients without stratification for other prognostic factors whose treatment was confined to alkylating agents. Modern prognostic factors, IgVH mutations, CD38 expression or ZAP-70 expression, now enable us to recognise a group of patients unlikely to need treatment in the next 25 years, and another group whose disease is likely to prove fatal within 8 years. Furthermore, we now have a series of treatments capable of inducing a molecular remission, even in advanced disease. The time has therefore arrived, Hamblin feels, to initiate controlled trials testing the hypothesis that poor prognosis CLL might be curable if treated early enough. In this context, the UK CLL Forum is about to begin two pilot studies looking at the possibility of achieving molecular remissions with treatment regimens involving a combination of fludarabine and cyclophosphamide together with either rituximab or alemtuzumab and further information on the conception and results of such studies are awaited with much interest by colleagues in the field.

We move, in Chapters Six and Seven, to a detailed documentation of current scientific evidence and expert opinion for the first and second line management of CLL. Alkylating agents alone or in combination were the standard treatment during the last decades and the advent of the purine analogues in the early 1990s, in particular fludarabine phosphate, had a major impact on the management of CLL. In first line therapy, as Cazin discusses in Chapter Six, fludarabine allows a higher response rate and a longer progression-free survival compared to CAP or to chlorambucil. Indeed, fludarabine is quite possibly the most active single agent in

CLL given its ability to achieve overall response rates (ORRs) of 63 to 70% and complete remission (CR) rates of 35%. Importantly, fludarabine has demonstrated its ability to improve the quality and duration of life in CLL, justifying its position in first-line therapy. In this context, it is useful that an oral formulation of fludarabine has been developed with an efficacy that appears not to differ from its intravenous formulation and with a safety profile that is essentially similar.

Fludarabine inhibits repair of DNA damage caused by agents such as mitoxantrone and cyclophosphamide which cause direct DNA damage and this synergistic effect has been demonstrated *in vitro* and confirmed *in vivo*. The response rate and progression-free survival with combination therapy are higher than with fludarabine alone, but no randomized trial has yet been published to confirm this observation. Oral combination therapy of cyclophosphamide and fludarabine in a 5 day regimen in untreated CLL patients has demonstrated a high response rate (80% ORR, 49.3 CR) but despite the high remission rate and long disease-free survival, chemotherapy alone is not curative for CLL and almost all patients have detectable MRD after the end of therapy and virtually all will experience a relapse. Complementary treatments targeted at eradicating MRD may, as Cazin describes, lead to improved outcomes. Indeed, the possibilities offered by intensification with high dose chemotherapy/radiotherapy with autologous stem cells support and above all (non-myeloablative) allogeneic stem cell transplantation, allow us to shift increasingly the focus from palliation to cure. Newer treatment approaches with monoclonal antibodies, while improving response rates and survival duration, do not appear curative. Rituximab administered concurrently with fludarabine in previously untreated patients demonstrates a better efficacy compared to sequential use and the combination of fludarabine, cyclophosphamide and rituximab leads to high response rates (66% CR) and a molecular response. Other clinical trials will study the benefit of consolidation therapy with alemtuzumab and the results of these studies are awaited with much interest. Randomized trials are required before retaining these combination therapies as standard treatment in younger patients but in the elderly, the choice of first line therapy needs to pay greater attention to potential toxicity and as a consequence classical treatments with chlorambucil or fludarabine alone may be indicated.

There have been no large randomised studies comparing treatments for patients with relapsed or refractory CLL and as Johnson, writing in Chapter Seven points out, evidence of benefit is based on historical control data and the results of randomised trials of initial treatment in which patients who fail to respond to one arm of the study are crossed over to another arm. The response to second line treatments depends on a variety of factors including clinical stage, adverse biological prognostic factors, the number of prior therapies and critically refractoriness to the last treatment and this author proceeds to detail and discuss our current knowledge in this context in this important chapter which closes Part Two of the volume.

We have dedicated Part Three of the volume to a consideration of further treatment strategies in CLL, namely stem-cell transplantation, the place of newer agents in development and trial for disease management and the treatment of immunodeficiency and autoimmune disease. Stem cell transplantation, as Milligan discusses in Chapter Eight, may be attractive for some younger patients with advanced CLL, offering them the opportunity of improved outcomes compared with standard treatment. Neither autologous nor allogeneic transplantation can be regarded as "standard of care" for patients with CLL and the author is clear that, where possible, patients with CLL undergoing a stem cell transplant should be enrolled into clinical trials. There have been no randomised studies of autologous transplantation in CLL. Early studies from Boston using purged bone marrow and a cyclophosphamide/TBI regimen demonstrated that the majority of patients became PCR negative for evidence of residual disease post autograft and 63% remained disease free after 4 years with an overall survival of 85%. The TRM was 10%. The UK MRC CLL pilot study has shown that about 50% of newly diagnosed patients can undergo a stem cell autograft with the principal reasons for failing to get a transplant being failure to achieve an adequate disease response to initial therapy or an inability to mobilise sufficient stem cells. In this study, 80% of patients became PCR negative post-autograft, but post-transplant monitoring showed that about half of these had evidence of molecular disease activity within 30 months. The clinical disease free survival at 5 years was 62% and OS 84% . The early transplant related mortality was 1.6 %, but of 62 patients transplanted 5 have shown evidence of tMDS. Further information, which Milligan describes, comes from the EBMT. In a study of over 300 transplants reported to the Registry, the TRM was 6% and 83% of patients were alive at 2 years. Favourable prognostic indicators were complete remission at the time of transplant and the use of TBI in the conditioning schedule. The German CLL 3 study has shown that patients with mutated V_H genes fare better after autograft. The clinical value of autografting may well be answered by the ongoing MRC CLL5/EBMT trial.

In terms of allogeneic transplantation, there exists a real potential for cure, as Milligan points out. Indeed, the TRM of earlier studies was unacceptable and has focused interest on newer RIC techniques although the long-term results of RIC transplants in CLL remain unknown. In a recent retrospective analysis by the EBMT comparing RIC with standard transplants in CLL, for example, the 2 year TRM was 22% v 33% and OS 68% versus 59%, respectively. Cox analysis showed an advantage for RIC v standard transplant for TRM (HR 0.5 [0.3-0.83]; p = 0.007) and OS (HR 0.56 [0.37–0.86]; p = 0.007) and longer-term follow up is therefore needed to define the place and timing of allogeneic transplantation in CLL.

As part of the intensive research activity for new treatment strategies in CLL, rapid, high-throughput analysis of thousands of novel compounds for therapeutic efficacy is now possible in routine drug development strategies, but the application of such methods to CLL is compromised not only by our lack of knowledge about the key molecules and pathways involved in the pathogenesis of CLL, but also by the lack of suitable *in vitro* models for the disease. Despite or because of these problems, a bewildering array of new agents and approaches are being developed, if not specifically for CLL then for the malignancies of mature B-cells in general, and it is to a stimulating discussion of these that Dyer turns in Chapter Nine. Different classes of compounds including proteasome inhibitors, inhibitors of various protein kinases such as PI-3 kinase, protein kinase C and cyclin dependent kinases, and inhibitors of histone deacetylases are now in clinical trial. The efficacy of antisense oligonucleotides to down-regulate the anti-apoptotic protein BCL2, has been assessed in a phase III study and these important results are awaited with much interest. Various monoclonal antibodies are also being assessed alone, in combination with each other, and with chemotherapy. The CD20 MAb, for example, has little activity on its own, but appears to synergise with fludarabine-based regimens, possibly through activation of pro-apoptotic molecules. HLADR MAbs may be of interest since they induce apoptosis via a caspase-independent mechanism. Second generation MAbs with enhanced binding to Fc receptors may have enhanced efficacy. However, none of the above approaches are specific for CLL. More genuinely targeted therapy should come from a better understanding of signalling pathways such as SDF1/CXCR4, IL4 *etc* involved in the maintenance of CLL viability *in vivo*, and possibly through identification of the CLL "stem cells".

Infection is a major cause of morbidity and mortality in patients with B cell chronic lymphocytic leukaemia. The majority of infectious episodes are due to bacterial infections, particularly of the upper respiratory tract but the incidence of viral infection is also increased, with herpes zoster representing a particular problem. Several factors contribute to this state of immunodeficiency, most notably hypogammaglobulinaemia and impaired cellular immune function and it is to the prophylaxis and management of infective complications of CLL that Moss turns in Chapter Ten. The management of hypogammaglobulinaemia is associated with impaired survival in B-CLL and its frequency increases with duration of disease. Impaired T cell and natural killer cell function is more difficult to quantitate, although several studies which the author discusses have shown abnormalities in phenotype and function. Although patients may be immunosuppressed in the early phase of their disease, this is much more apparent with advanced disease and particularly following treatment and a recent study which Moss highlights has shown that the number of previous chemotherapy regimens is the major determinant of infectious episodes.

Approaches to control infectious disease may be applied either to all patients or targeted to those at particular risk, such as patients with heavily pre-treated disease. Early awareness and prompt treatment of any infectious complication, as Moss emphasises, is a mainstay of supportive care. Prophylactic antibiotic usage is less widely employed with the exception of co-trimoxazole prophylaxis following the use of purine analogues. Intravenous immunoglobulin has been used for patients with hypogammaglobulinaemia and randomised trials have shown a significant reduction in infectious episodes. Unfortunately, however, these benefits are rarely cost-effective and there is little evidence for prolongation of life. The increasing use of intensive chemotherapy and monoclonal antibodies can lead to profound immunosuppression and appropriate prophylactic procedures must be in place.

Having considered the problem of serious infection in CLL we move to a consideration of the autoimmune complications which may arise as part of the disease process. Autoimmunity, as Hamblin points out within Chapter Eleven, has long been recognised as a complication of CLL, but how this comes about is largely misunderstood. Because the CD5 positive B1 cell in the mouse has been associated with autoimmunity in certain inbred species, and because the surface immunoglobulin of CLL cells exhibits a certain 'stickiness' that could be interpreted as immune reactivity against a range of autoantigens related to phospholipids, it has been assumed that CLL is a tumour of B1 cells and that the immunoglobulin it produces, being autoreactive, is the cause of autoimmune disease. Hamblin is clear that, in fact, neither of these assumptions is true. Autoimmune haemolytic anaemia (AIHA) occurs in about 10% of cases of CLL and the autoantibody is not the product of the tumour (except very rarely in cold haemagglutination syndrome), but of the residual normal B cells. It is most likely, as the author points out, to occur in patients with long-standing, multiply treated disease, and may be triggered by treatment, especially with fludarabine, though it may also occur as a presenting feature of CLL. Immune thrombocytopenia occurs in about 2% of cases, often in similar circumstances to AIHA and sometimes together. Other types of autoimmune disease are very rare in CLL, indeed the only types that can be said with certainty to occur more commonly in CLL than in age matched controls are autoimmune neutropenia, pure red cell aplasia, paraneoplastic pemphigus, nephrotic syndrome and acquired angio-oedema. Treatment follows conventional guidelines, but AIHA following fludarabine is especially severe, often requiring cyclosporine or rituximab to control it.

No volume on CLL would be complete without a proper consideration of the nature and progress of ongoing and planned clinical trials aimed at the generation of *new knowledge* for disease management, and of progress in the development of clinical practice guidelines aimed at codifying *existing knowledge* with the aim of providing optimal care to the patient with CLL. We have therefore committed the final part of the volume, Part Four, to a review of progress in these particular contexts. In Chapter Twelve, Catovsky, on behalf of the CLL Working Group and the Adult Leukaemia Working Party of the National Cancer Research Institute, provides a detailed overview of the principal randomized studies of treatments for CLL that have been conducted over the last twenty years. The largest of these, CLL4, has, as the author describes, been running for four and a half years and had exceeded its target of 500 patients at the time of writing. Recruitment will continue, Catovsky confirms, for another two years with a new target of 750. Important characteristics of CLL4 are its particular clinical, scientific and quality of life objectives which will produce a large amount of new data about prognostic groups in CLL and their response to therapy. The main comparison is between chlorambucil (at $70mg/m^2/month$, which is almost double the dose used in other studies), fludarabine (oral or IV) and the combination fludarabine + cyclophosphamide (oral or IV).

In comparison with previous trials, CLL1, 2 and 3, the overall responses in CLL4 are higher and the current projected survival also appears better. One striking point seen in CLL4 (and all other trials) is the better survival of females with CLL. In an analysis of 1379 patients randomised in CLL1, 2, 3 and 4, 25% of females had CR against 22% of males, and 21% were non-responders, in contrast to 29.4% of males ($p = 0.006$). Previous trials have also identified stage, age and response as important prognostic variables. However, stage is only significant if it includes all CLL patients, not just those who need therapy. The survival of stage A progressive patients in both CLL3 and 4 is similar to that of stage B patients. Survival is an important outcome in CLL and generally response to therapy correlates with survival. However, as CLL patients may respond to first, second or third line therapy, their survival improves with each good response; thus, progression free survival may be a better indication of effectiveness of a given therapy. In CLL4, survival by response is not yet significant, but progression free survival already shows a clear trend for the good responders (CR and nodular PR versus PR).

The toxicities in CLL4 that Catovsky describes are as expected: more neutropenia (53%) with fludarabine + cyclophosphamide than with fludarabine (42%) or chlorambucil (32%) alone and this correlates with slightly more febrile episodes. Nausea and vomiting are also greater with the fludarabine + cyclophosphamide combination, as well as alopecia. The availability of new agents, such as the antibodies rituximab and Campath-1H, offer an exciting prospect of better and newer combinations in CLL therapy. There are interesting results with high dose methylprednisolone in resistant CLL and with the combination of fludarabine, cyclophosphamide and mitozantrone (FCM), which also showed promise in a Spanish and German series. CLL4 is not just about initial therapy, as Catovsky emphasises. An important component is the second randomisation to use results from in-vitro testing (the DiSC assay) and a quality of life questionnaire. Laboratory studies include FISH analysis with five probes to test the hierarchical model of Dohner, VH mutation status, CD38 and ZAP testing by flow cytometry. The results of these studies will have a major impact in selecting prognostic groups to be assessed against new treatment modalities beyond CLL4.

Clinical practice guidelines represent one of many means for enhancing the translation of new knowledge into routine clinical practice and it is to guidelines for the investigation and management of CLL that Oscier and Johnson turn in Chapter Thirteen, the closing chapter of this volume. The CLL guidelines, as these authors discuss, have been compiled by the Guidelines Working Group of the UK CLL Forum at the request of the Haemato-Oncology Task Force of the British Committee for Standards in Haematology (BCSH), a Committee of the British Society for Haematology (BSH). The Working Group was constituted with representation from haematology and oncology and included a patient representative. Draft guidelines were reviewed by members of the UK CLL Forum, patient representatives, members of the BCSH and a panel of UK haematologists. The comments were incorporated where appropriate into an interim guideline which was later formally published following peer-review in the British Journal of Haematology. The guidelines, as Oscier and Johnson describe, cover the diagnostic criteria for CLL, the use of prognostic markers, indications for referral of patients from primary to secondary care, patient information, indications for treatment and assessment of response, a treatment strategy for CLL for both untreated and previously treated patients and the management of complications such as infections, auto-immune cytopenias and lymphomatous transformation. Importantly, and in order to ensure the incorporation of continuously evolving knowledge, a full guideline revision is planned for 2007.

In this volume we have aimed to provide a synthesis of current knowledge on the investigation and management of chronic lymphocytic leukaemia that is as concise as possible but as detailed as necessary. Consultants and non-consultant career grades in haematology and medical and clinical oncology are likely to find it of particular use as part of continuing professional development studies and we advance the book explicitly as an excellent resource for this purpose. We anticipate, in addition, that the book will prove of very considerable interest and use to clinical nurse specialists and oncology pharmacists working in these specialties and to the commissioners, planners and managers of cancer services as part of their own individual responsibilities for the provision of an effective clinical service. Finally, we thank Schering Health Care Ltd for the award of the grant of unrestricted educational sponsorship that enabled the organisation of a national symposium on the investigation and management of CLL with the UK CLL Forum, the Association of Cancer Physicians and The Royal College of Radiologists at The Royal College of Pathologists, London, at which synopses of the individual chapters of this book were presented.

Terry Hamblin DM FRCP FRCPath FMedSci
Stephen Johnson MB BS FRCP FRCPath
Andrew Miles MSc MPhil PhD

London, October 2004

PART 1

Genetics and natural history

Chapter 1

Familial chronic lymphocytic leukaemia

Gabrielle Sellick, Daniel Catovsky and Richard S. Houlston

Introduction

In Western countries, leukaemia affects about 1–2% of the population (Miller *et al.* 1993) B-cell chronic lymphocytic leukaemia (CLL) is the most common form of leukaemia, accounting for approximately 30% of all cases (Gale & Foon 1987). Acute leukaemia occurs at a higher frequency in individuals with constitutional chromosome anomalies and is a feature of several Mendelian cancer syndromes. Although such associations are well established, inherited susceptibility has not, until recently, been recognized in CLL and other related B-cell lymphoproliferative disorders (LPDs). Evidence from large epidemiological and family studies, however, strongly supports the notion that a subset of CLL involves inherited susceptibility. Identification of genes predisposing to CLL will be useful for future diagnosis and treatment of the disease, as well as for helping elucidate the underlying events leading to B-cell tumorigenesis in general. Here we review the current status of knowledge about inherited susceptibility to CLL.

Evidence for genetic predisposition to chronic lymphocytic leukaemia

Over 50 families have been reported in the literature who show distinct clustering of CLL (Yuille *et al.* 2000a). It has often been suggested that even very striking familial clusters of common malignancies can be ascribed to ascertainment bias. This is a statistical fallacy: for example, a family with three siblings affected with CLL would be expected to occur by chance about every 1,000 years in England. Hence striking multiple-case families provide very strong evidence for an increased familial risk. In addition, several large families have been reported who show vertical transmission of CLL and other LPDs, suggesting that predisposition to CLL and other LPDs is caused by the inheritance of a dominantly acting gene (or genes) with incomplete penetrance and pleiotropic effects (Yuille *et al.* 2000a).

Eight epidemiological studies have systematically examined the risk for the development of CLL and other LPDs in relatives of patients (Gunz *et al.* 1975; Giles *et al.* 1984; Cartwright *et al.* 1987; Linet *et al.* 1989; Pottern *et al.* 1991; Goldgar *et al.* 1994; Radovanovic *et al.* 1994; Goldin *et al.* 2003) (Table 1.1). All have reported elevated risks of CLL in relatives. The study reported by Goldin and Hemminki (2003) is the largest and most informative so far (Goldin *et al.* 2003). This study was based on around 6,000 CLL cases within the Swedish family cancer database. In addition to a 7-fold increase in risk of CLL in first-degree relatives, risks of other LPDs were also shown to be elevated (Table 1.1) (Goldin *et al.* 2003).

Table 1.1 Familial relative risks of CLL and other LPDs

Study	Index case		Relative risk (95% CI)
Cohort studies			
Gunz *et al.* (1975)	Leukaemia	Leukaemia in first-degree relatives	2.4 (1.9–3.9)
Giles *et al.* (1984)	LPD	LPD in first-degree relatives	3.4 (2.4–4.7)
Goldgar *et al.* (1994)	Lymphocytic leukaemia	Lymphocytic leukaemias in first-degree relatives	5.7 (2.6–10.0)
Case-control studies			
Cartwright *et al.* (1987)	CLL	Lymphocytic leukaemias	4.3 (0.9–19.5)
Linet *et al.* (1989)	CLL	Leukaemia in parents and siblings	2.6 (1.2–5.5)
Pottern *et al.* (1991)	CLL	Leukaemia in parents and siblings	2.3 (1.2–4.4)
Radovanovic *et al.* (1994)	CLL	Leukaemia in first- and second-degree relatives	
Goldin & Hemminki (2003)	CLL	CLL in first-degree relatives	7.5 (3.9–14.6)
	CLL	Non-Hodgkin's lymphoma in first-degree relatives	1.5 (1–2.2)
	CLL	Hodgkin's lymphoma in first-degree relatives	2.4 (1.1–5.1)

Characteristics of familial chronic lymphocytic leukaemia

The phenotype of earlier age of onset and increased risk of second tumours is a classical feature of many familial cancers. One recent survey of the clinical features of 28 CLL families containing 73 cases suggests that familial cases present about 10 years earlier than sporadic cases, implying a more aggressive clonal expansion (Ishibe *et al.* 2001). A higher frequency of second primary tumours, but not large-cell non-Hodgkin's lymphoma (Richter's syndrome), has also been reported. One intriguing feature seen in the expression of CLL in many of the families reported is anticipation, the phenomenon of earlier onset and more severe phenotype in successive generations (Pottern *et al.* 1991; Horwitz *et al.* 1996; Yuille *et al.* 1998; Goldin *et al.* 1999; Wiernik *et al.* 2001). The age at diagnosis in offspring of those affected appears to be about 10–20 years earlier than in the parental generation. There is, however, a caveat to deriving information about clinical phenotypes from families ascertained for research as these tend to be enriched for young cases, potentially introducing bias through censoring or cohort effects.

It is probable that familial CLL is genetically heterogeneous. Two studies have determined immunoglobulin V (IgV) status in familial cases (Pritsch *et al.* 1999; Sakai *et al.* 2000). Whereas the distribution of phenotypes in the families reported by Pritsch *et al* (1999) was not significantly different from that expected (on the basis of the observed prevalence of the mutated phenotype), the distribution in the families reported by Sakai *et al.* (2000) shows a deviation. Combining data from the two studies, the inter-familial concordance between those affected is significant, suggesting that assessing IgV status may be helpful in sub-group analyses in searches for susceptibility alleles for CLL.

Although most families reported so far are nuclear, it is conceivable that many apparently unaffected family members have sub-clinical CLL if the lifetime risk conferred by a disease allele is less than 30%. Monoclonal B-cells with CLL-phenotype are detectable in about 3% of the population by using a sensitive flow cytometric analysis of CD5/CD20/CD79b expression on CD19-gated B cells (Rawstron *et al.* 2002a). The absolute cell numbers are on average 1000-fold lower than the levels required for a clinical diagnosis of CLL. To determine whether this CLL-phenotype reflects an inherited predisposition, we examined 59 healthy, first-degree relatives of CLL patients from 21 families (Rawstron *et al.* 2002b). Cells with a CLL-phenotype were detected in eight (13.5%) relatives representing a significant over representation (Figure 1.1) (Rawstron *et al.* 2002a, b). CLL-phenotype cell levels were stable over time as shown by sequential analysis and had the characteristics of indolent CLL (low CD38 expression) (Rawstron *et al.* 2002c). However, indolent and aggressive clinical disease forms were present in the familial index cases suggesting that initiation and proliferation of the disease may involve different biological processes. Recently, Marti *et al.* (2003) presented similar findings, confirming our initial observation. Follow-up studies are clearly required to determine the incidence of the B-cell monoclonal phenotype and its relationship to both CLL and B-cell LPD disease progression.

Models of inherited predisposition

So far, little is known about the identity of the genes conferring susceptibility to CLL. However, as previously mentioned, epidemiological studies show the risk for first-degree relatives of CLL cases, averaged across all ages, is increased 7-fold. Most of this familial risk is probably genetic in origin. Such moderate/high familial risks are entirely compatible with a wide range of allele frequencies and penetrances (Table 1.2).

Large published pedigrees support the existence of mutations conferring a high risk of disease (high penetrance susceptibility alleles). Such mutations may cause a substantial proportion of young age-onset cases and large multiple-case families

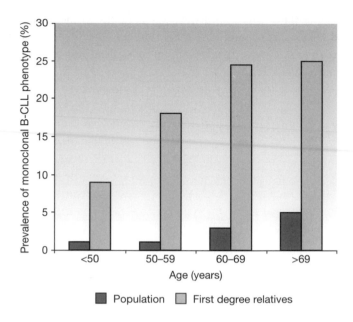

Figure 1.1 Prevalence of monoclonal B-CLL phenotype in relatives of familial CLL index cases compared with the general population.

Table 1.2 Models of genetic susceptibility that could account for the increased familial risk in CLL (note the real situation is unknown)

	RR	Frequency of allele in population	Number of alleles required to account for a familial relative risk of 7.5*
High penetrance allele	25	0.002	3–7†
Low penetrance allele	4	0.01	27–83
	4	0.1	8–24
	4	0.3	13–41

*Lower figure is based on the assumption that alleles interact multiplicatively (i.e. the penetrance of the disease is the product of the penetrances contributed by two or more loci); upper figure assumes that alleles interact additively (i.e. the penetrance of the disease is represented by the sum of the penetrances contributed by two or more loci). †Realistically in the scenario of high penetrance gene mutation, only the additive model is appropriate approximating to locus heterogeneity.

(Figure 1.2) but are unlikely to be responsible for a similar proportion of cases in the elderly population. Low penetrance variants conferring more modest risks, typically of about 2–4 may also make an important contribution to overall familial risk. There may be many such alleles, which individually have small effects, but when taken together contribute significantly to disease susceptibility in the general population. More than 80 such variants could contribute to susceptibility, each independently conferring a small risk but acting additively or multiplicatively to cause a very high risk in a few individuals (Table 1.2).

Highly penetrant or moderately penetrant mutations giving rise to large multi-generational families can be detected through genetic linkage. The number of families required to identify low penetrance alleles by linkage is, however, prohibitively large (typically over 2,000). In contrast, the sample size required to identify low-penetrance genes based on allelic association can be much smaller (Risch & Merikangas 1996). Whereas polymorphisms in several candidate genes have been evaluated as low penetrance predisposition loci for CLL, so far many of the reported studies are based on small sample sizes and hence the robustness of these findings are questionable. Association studies based on unselected cases are satisfactory for the evaluation of common variants but have limited power if the carrier frequency of the deleterious allele is less than 5% (Houlston & Peto 2003). The power of association studies can, however, be greatly enhanced by using cases selected for a family history of the disease (Risch & Merikangas 1996). In addition, the detection of CLL-phenotype cells may provide a surrogate marker of carrier status, potentially enhancing gene identification through mapping in families and direct analysis of isolated CLL-phenotype cells.

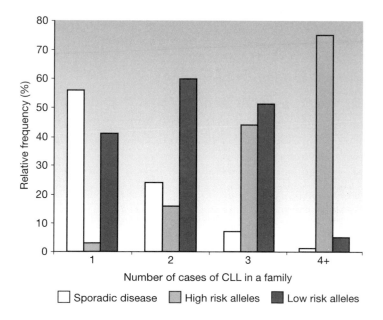

Figure 1.2 Contribution of low- and high-risk alleles to the incidence of familial CLL.

Detection of susceptibility alleles causing chronic lymphocytic leukaemia

Little is known about the genetic basis of CLL. The search for predisposition genes is currently restricted to the evaluation of a limited number of candidates for which there is *a priori* evidence suggesting involvement in disease onset and progression.

One strategy for identifying novel susceptibility loci is to undertake whole genome linkage analysis of multiple-case families. So far, only one such study based on 18 families has been performed, with six regions identified on chromosomes 1, 3, 6, 12, 13 and 17 achieving LOD (logarithm of the odds) scores of around 1.0 (Goldin *et al.* 2003). The authors failed to find any genomic regions that achieved statistical significance. Much larger linkage studies are required if allelic heterogeneity is assumed to be present in the aetiology of CLL.

Another strategy for identifying disease susceptibility alleles in the absence of large multi-case families is to define regions of recurrent genomic loss in tumour cells from familial cases. The technique of comparative genomic hybridization (CGH) allows this type of investigation by examining the whole genome for regions of chromosomal loss or gain. We have applied CGH to 24 familial cases of CLL. Chromosome losses documented frequently in sporadic CLL were observed at a comparable frequency in the familial cases analysed (e.g. 11q23 and 13q14) (Summersgill *et al.* 2002). In addition, the data indicated that three regions of the genome might harbour predisposition genes on the basis of notable allelic imbalance: Xp11.2-p21, Xq21-qter, 2p12-p14 and 4q11-q21. Considerable caution is called for in extrapolating from CGH data, and only detailed investigation of these regions of the genome will allow candidate familial CLL gene identification.

Candidate CLL predisposition genes

The ataxia telangiectasia mutated (ATM) gene

Several chromosomal breakage syndromes have been known for many years to be associated with an increased risk of leukaemia (German 1980) including the recessive disease, ataxia telangiectasia (A-T). A-T patients have an increased risk of lymphoma and leukaemia (Taylor *et al.* 1996; Olsen *et al.* 2001) CLL has also been reported in A-T families suggesting that A-T heterozygotes may be at an increased risk. In a retrospective study of the cancer incidence in 110 A-T families, the risk of haematological and lymphoid malignancies was increased in blood relatives of A-T patients. CLL accounted for all but one of the leukaemias seen in the adult blood relatives although these observations did not attain formal statistical significance (Swift *et al* 1987).

ATM is mutated in about 20% of CLL samples, and some patients have been reported to harbour germline mutations (Schaffner *et al.* 1999; Stankovic *et al.* 1999). Homozygous *ATM* germline mutations are associated with genomic instability and radiosensitivity conferring an increase in mutation rate and homologous recombination, mis-pairing double strand breaks and a high frequency of cytogenetic rearrangements. A-T cells also show defects in cell cycle checkpoints. The cellular role of ATM and the prevalence of leukaemia in relatives of A-T patients have led researchers to question whether germline *ATM* mutations confer an increased risk of CLL. We assessed the role of ATM in familial CLL through a linkage analysis of 28 families (Bevan *et al.* 1999). The distribution of sharing of *ATM* haplotypes between affected individuals did not lend support to the notion that *ATM* is involved in familial CLL. However, the study was not sufficiently empowered to preclude that *ATM* might account for up to a 2-fold sibling relative risk. It is conceivable that genes conferring susceptibility to CLL are associated with more modest risks. Two studies have directly assessed the contribution of *ATM* to CLL by DNA sequence analysis. The first of these studies was reported by Stankovic *et al.* (1999) who observed two germline ATM mutations in 32 cases (6.3%) of CLL. One of the mutations identified was a truncating mutation, the other a missense mutation (P1054R)—which the authors designated as pathogenic. The observation of two mutations in 32 cases is significant. P1054R has, however, been designated as a polymorphism by some workers. We have recently assessed the contribution of *ATM* to CLL predisposition through an analysis of 61 cases derived from 29 families (Yuille *et al.* 2002). Two cases of different familial origin were found to have truncating *ATM* mutations; however, one was clearly somatic. In addition, several missense changes were detected, including C4258T and C6919T. Although C4258T has previously been reported as a mutation causing A-T, it is difficult to assign pathogenicity to many missense changes in the absence of robust functional assays for each domain of the gene.

The contribution of *ATM* to CLL predisposition depends critically on the carrier frequency of pathogenic mutations in the general population. Most estimates derived from the population prevalence of A-T suggest a carrier frequency of about 1% (Easton 1994). Existing data, therefore, appear to suggest an over-representation of *ATM* mutations in CLL. However, it seems unlikely that such mutations represent a major susceptibility locus for the disease as the familial relative risk ascribable to mutations is unlikely to be more than about 1.1 (Yuille *et al.* 2002).

The major histocompatability complex (MHC)

The established relationship between human leukocyte antigen (HLA) and Hodgkin's lymphoma, another B-cell disorder, and the association between autoimmune disease and CLL raises the possibility that genes within the MHC region may be determinants of CLL susceptibility. Hodgkin's lymphoma shows strong linkage to HLA (Risch 1987). The underlying basis of linkage is, however, not through a restricted haplotype: rather, it appears that a range of HLA-DPB1 alleles affect susceptibility or resistance to specific subtypes of Hodgkin's lymphoma (Klitz *et al.* 1994). Intriguingly, CLL patients frequently share common HLA haplotypes with relatives who have autoimmune disease. Hence genetic determinants of CD5$^+$ B-cell proliferation or differentiation are likely to be involved in both B-CLL and autoimmune disease. The notion of a relationship between CLL and autoimmune disease is supported by animal studies using congenic New Zealand mouse strains (Okada *et al.* 1991; Hirose *et al.* 1997). In Hodgkin's disease the allele sharing probabilities between affected siblings suggest that the HLA locus is likely to explain a two-fold sibling relative risk with more than half of all cases arising in susceptible individuals. There is no evidence such a situation exists for familial CLL. In the linkage study reported by Bevan *et al.* (2000) there was no evidence for linkage in an analysis of 27 families. However, the 95% confidence limit for the estimate of the sibling relative risk ascribable to the HLA did not preclude that variation within HLA or the MHC is a determinant of CLL susceptibility. A case–control study of 101 CLL patients and 157 controls has recently reported a significantly increased frequency of HLA-DRB4*0103 (relative risk (RR), 2.8) (Machulla *et al.* 2001). The presence of alleles HLA-DRB1*0401, HLA-DQB1*0302 and HLA-DPB1*0301, as well as of homozygosity for HLA-DQB1, was also associated with a higher risk for CLL, albeit non-significantly. Haplotype analysis showed a CLL-specific linkage disequilibrium for HLA-DRB1*0401: DRB4*0103 and HLA-DRB4*0103:DQB1*0302. Although these findings suggest that CLL may be associated with the HLA-DR-DR53-DQ8 haplotype, which has been previously associated with several auto-immune diseases, further studies are required to determine the robustness of this suggested association.

The B-cell antigen receptor complex (BCR)

The BCR comprises membrane immunoglobulins (mIgs) and a heterodimer of Ig (CD79a) and Ig (CD79b) transmembrane proteins, encoded by the MB-1 and B29 genes, respectively (Payelle-Brogard *et al.* 1999). These proteins are necessary for surface expression of mIg and BCR signaling. CLL B-cells frequently express low to undetectable surface Ig, as well as CD79b protein and show abnormal B29 expression and/or function. The possibility that these abnormalities might be a consequence of *B29* mutations has been assessed in a study of 10 CLL families (Payelle-Brogard *et al.* 1999). Although a few silent or replacement mutations were observed, none led to a truncated CD79b protein; furthermore, there was no evidence of co-segregation of mutation with disease, strongly implying that germline mutations in *B29* are unlikely to cause familial CLL.

The P2X7 receptor gene

It has been suggested that a predisposing factor for CLL might be an inherited failure of mechanisms involved in apoptosis of lymphocytes. Activation of the P2X7 receptor leads to apoptosis of lymphocytes in individuals with CLL, and reduced function of this receptor has an anti-apoptotic effect, resulting in an increase in B-cell numbers. Inheritance of a loss-of-function polymorphic variant at position 1513 in the P2X7 gene has recently been associated with the pathogenesis of CLL (Wiley *et al.* 2002).

In a study of 36 CLL cases and 46 controls the prevalence of the *P2X7* 1513 A>C polymorphism was reported to be higher in cases than in controls (odds ratio 5.3; 95% CI 1.8–15.7) (Wiley *et al.* 2002). Furthermore, in two CLL families – a father/son pair and a sister/sister pair with CLL – loss of P2X7 function appeared to be a consequence of the inheritance of one or two 1513C alleles. As the population frequency of the C allele is about 8%, the associated 5.3-fold increase in risk translates to a sibling relative risk of 1.4 (assuming a dominant model), thereby accounting for a significant portion of the overall familial risk. Association studies are, however, capricious if based on small numbers, as illustrated recently by data from two additional studies, both of which failed to provide evidence of a link between CLL incidence and P2X7 1513 A/C genotype when using larger sample numbers (Thunberg *et al.* 2002; Ibbotson *et al.* 2003). One study did, however, show the polymorphism was correlated with patient survival, although only when individuals were adjusted for mutated VH status (Thunberg *et al.* 2002).

The role of trinucleotide repeat expansion

In several Mendelian diseases anticipation has been shown to be indicative of a dynamic mutation mechanism involving expansion of a triplet repeat motif (Ashley & Warren 1995). To examine the possibility that nucleotide repeat expansion is a feature of familial CLL, the repeat expansion detection (RED) technique has recently been applied to samples from 17 patients with familial disease and 32 patients with early-onset CLL (Benzow *et al.* 2002). No potentially pathological CAG expansions were detected. Accepting the caveat that the expansion may be outside the detection limit for RED, the finding suggests that such expansions are not a key feature of CLL. Other processes that may be involved in generating anticipation include a cohort effect in relation to viral or other environmental exposures that act as risk factors.

Other genes

Linkage of Hodgkin's disease to the pseudo-autosomal region of the genome has been proposed by Horwitz & Wiernik (1999) on the basis of an excess of sex concordance among affected siblings. The common lineage of Hodgkin's and CLL prompted us to examine whether familial CLL also shows pseudo-autosomal linkage. An analysis of 75 CLL families showed that the frequency of sex-concordant sib pairs is skewed beyond random expectation (Yuille *et al.* 2000b). However, it is impossible to preclude publication bias and so the implicated pseudo-autosomal linkage in CLL so far is questionable.

Conclusions

Among all haematological malignancies, B-cell CLL has the highest familial clustering (three- to sevenfold increase), which is strongly suggestive of the existence of inherited predisposition to CLL and other associated B-cell LPDs. It is probable that in addition to alleles conferring a significant genetic risk part of the inherited susceptibility to the disease is mediated through numerous low-risk alleles. Importantly, the identification of the genes involved in familial forms of CLL should provide insights into the pathogenesis of CLL in general. At present there is no compelling evidence that any specific gene acts as a major susceptibility locus. The future identification of genes conferring CLL susceptibility will depend upon a combination of dense genome-wide linkage studies and highly empowered association studies. Experience in the study of other familial cancers has shown that the ascertainment and collection of families necessary for such studies is only achievable through multi-centre collaborations. To expedite collection of CLL families we have formed a linkage consortium.

Acknowledgements

The authors' work is supported by the Leukaemia Research Fund and the Kay Kendall Trust.

References

Ashley, C. T. & Warren, S. T. (1995). Trinucleotide repeat expansion and human disease. *Annual Review of Genetics* **29**, 703–728.

Benzow, K. A., Koob, M. D., Condie, A., Catovsky, D., Matutes, E., Yuille, M. R. & Houlston, R. S. (2002). Instability of CAG-trinucleotide repeats in chronic lymphocytic leukaemia. *Leukemia and Lymphoma* **43**, 1987–1990.

Bevan, S., Catovsky, D., Marossy, A., Popat, S., Antonvic, P., Bell, A., Ben-Bassat, I., Berrebi, A., Mauro, F., Pittion, A. and 9 others (1999). Linkage analysis for ATM in familial chronic lymphocytic leukaemia. *Leukaemia* **13**, 1497–1500.

Bevan, S., Catovsky, D., Matutes E., Antonovic P., Auger M. J., Ben-Bassat I., Bell, A., Berrebi, A., Gaminara, E. J., Mauro, F. R., and 11 others (2000). Linkage analysis for MHC related genetic susceptibility in familial chronic lymphocytic leukaemia. *Blood* **96**, 3982–3984.

Cartwright, R. A., Bernard, S. M., Bird, C. C., Darwin, C. M., O'Brien, C., Richards, I. D., Roberts, B. & McKinney, P. A. (1987). Chronic lymphocytic leukaemia: case–control epidemiological study in Yorkshire. *British Journal of Cancer* **56**, 79–82.

Easton, D. F. (1994). Cancer risks in A-T heterozygotes. *International Journal of Radiation Biology* **66**, S177–S182.

Gale, R. P. & Foon, K. A. (1987). Biology of chronic lyphocytic leukaemia. *Seminars in Haematology* **24**, 209–229.

German, J. (1980). Chromosome-breakage syndromes: different genes, different treatments, different cancers. *Basic Life Sciences* **15**, 429–439.

Giles, G. G., Lickiss, J. N., Baikie, M. J., Lowenthal, R. M. & Panton, J. J. (1984). Myeloproliferative and lymphoproliferative disorders in Tasmania, 1972–1980: occupational and familial aspects. *Journal of the National Cancer Institute* **72**, 1233–1124.

Goldgar, D. E., Easton, D. F., Cannon-Albright, L. A. & Skolnick, M. H. (1994). Systematic population-based assessment of cancer risk in first-degree relatives of cancer probands. *Journal of the National Cancer Institute* **86**, 1600–1608.

Goldin, L. R. & Hemminki, K. (2003). Familial risk of lymphoproliferative tumors in families of patients with chronic lymphocytic leukaemia: Results from the Swedish family-cancer database. *Leukemia and Lymphoma* **44**(Suppl. 2), 5.

Goldin, L. R., Ishibe, N., Sgambati, M., Marti, G. E., Fontaine, L., Lee, M. P., Kelley, J. M., Scherpbier, T., Buetow, K. H. & Caporaso, N. E. (2003). A genome scan of 18 families with chronic lymphocytic leukaemia. *British Journal of Haematology* **121**, 866–873.

Goldin, L. R., Sgambati, M., Marti, G. E., Fontaine, L., Ishibe, N. & Caporaso, N. (1999). Anticipation in familial chronic lymphocytic leukaemia. *American Journal of Human Genetics* **65**, 265–269.

Gunz, F. W., Gunz, J. P., Veale, A. M., Chapman, C. J. & Houston, I. B. (1975). Familial leukaemia: a study of 909 families. *Scandinavian Journal of Haematology* **15**, 117–131.

Hirose, S, Hamano, Y. & Shirai, T. (1997). Genetic factors predisposing to B-CLL and to autoimmune disease in spontaneous murine model. *Leukaemia* **11**(Suppl. 3), 267–270.

Horwitz, M., Goode, E. L. & Jarvik, G. P. (1996). Anticipation in familial leukaemia. *American Journal of Human Genetics* **59**, 990–998.

Horwitz, M. & Wiernik, P. H. (1999). Pseudoautosomal linkage of Hodgkin disease. *American Journal of Human Genetics* **65**, 1413–1422.

Houlston, R. S. & Peto, J. (2003). The future of association studies of common cancers. *Human Genetics* **112**, 434–435.

Ibbotson, R. E., Yan Zhang, L., Orchard, J. A., Oscier, D. G. & Cross, N. C. (2003). P2X7 polymorphism and chronic lymphocytic leukaemia:lack of correlation with incidence, survival and abnormalities of chromosome 12. *Leukemia and Lymphoma* **44**(Suppl. 2), 6.

Ishibe, N., Sgambati, M. T., Fontaine, L., Goldin, L. R., Jain, N., Weissman, N., Marti, G. E. & Caporaso, N. E. (2001). Clinical characteristics of familial B-CLL in the National Cancer Institute Familial Registry. *Leukemia and Lymphoma* **42**, 99–108.

Klitz, W., Aldrich, C. L., Fildes, N., Horning, S. J. & Begovich, A. B. (1994). Localization of predisposition to Hodgkin disease in the HLA class II region. *American Journal of Human Genetics* **54**, 497–505.

Hirose, S., Hamano, Y. & Shirai, T. (1997). Genetic factors predisposing to B-CLL and to autoimmune disease in spontaneous murine model. *Leukaemia* **11**(Suppl. 3), 267–270.

Linet, M. S., Van Natta, M. L., Brookmeyer, R., Khoury, M. J., McCaffrey, L. D., Humphrey, R. L. & Szklo, M. (1989). Familial cancer history and chronic lymphocytic leukaemia. A case–control study. *American Journal of Epidemiology* **130**, 655–664.

Machulla, H. K., Muller, L. P., Schaaf, A., Kujat, G., Schonermarck, U. & Langner, J. (2001). Association of chronic lymphocytic leukaemia with specific alleles of the HLA-DR4:DR53:DQ8 haplotype in German patients. *International Journal of Cancer* **92**, 203–207.

Marti, G. E., Carter, P., Abbasi, F., Washington, G. C., Jain, N., Zenger, V. E., Ishibe, N., Goldin, L., Fontaine, L., Weissman, N. and 8 others (2003). B-cell monoclonal lymphocytosis and B-cell abnormalities in the setting of familial B-cell chronic lymphocytic leukaemia. *Cytometry* **52B**, 1–12.

Miller, B. A., Ries, L. A. G., Hankey, B. F., Kosary, C. L., Harras, A. & Devesa, S. S. (1993). Cancer Statistics Review 1973–90, National Cancer Institute, National Institutes of Health Publication No. 93, 2789.

Okada, T., Takiura, F., Tokushige, K., Nozawa, S., Kiyosawa, T., Nakauchi, H., Hirose, S. & Shirai, T. (1991). Major histocompatibility complex controls clonal proliferation of CD5+ B cells in H-2-congenic New Zealand mice: a model for B cell chronic lymphocytic leukaemia and autoimmune disease. *European Journal of Immunology* **21**, 2743–2748.

Olsen, J.H., Hahnemann, J.M., Borresen-Dale, A.L., Brondum-Nielsen, K., Hammarstrom, L., Kleinerman, R., Kaariainen, H., Lonnqvist, T., Sankila, R., Seersholm, N. and 4 others (2001). Cancer in patients with ataxia-telangiectasia and in their relatives in the Nordic countries. *Journal of the National Cancer Institute* **93**, 121–127.

Payelle-Brogard, B., Magnac, C., Mauro, F. R., Mandelli, F., Dighiero, G. (1999). Analysis of the B-cell receptor B29 (CD79b) gene in familial chronic lymphocytic leukaemia. *Blood* **94**, 3516–3522.

Pottern, L. M., Linet, M., Blair, A., Dick, F., Burmeister, L. F., Gibson, R., Schuman, L. M. & Fraumeni, J. F. Jr (1991). Familial cancers associated with subtypes of leukamia and non-Hodgkin's lymphoma. *Leukaemia Research* **15**, 305–314.

Pritsch, O., Troussard, X., Magnac, C., Mauro, F.R., Davi, F., Payelle-Brogard, B., Dumas, G., Pulik, M., Clerget, F., Mandelli, F. and 4 others (1999). VH gene usage by family members affected with chronic lymphocytic leukaemia. *British Journal of Haematology* **107**, 616–624.

Radovanovic, Z., Markovic-Denic, L. & Jakovic, S. (1994). Cancer mortality of family members of patients with chronic lymphocytic leukaemia. *European Journal of Epidemiology* **10**, 211–213.

Rawstron, A. C., Green, M. J., Kuzmicki, A., Kennedy, B., Fenton, J. A., Evans, P. A., O'Connor, S. J., Richards, S. J., Morgan, G. J., Jack, A. S. & Hillmen, P. (2002a). Monoclonal B lymphocytes with the characteristics of "indolent" chronic lymphocytic leukaemia are present in 3.5% of adults with normal blood counts. *Blood* **100**, 635–639.

Rawstron, A. C., Yuille, M. R., Fuller, J., Cullen, M., Kennedy, B., Richards, S. J., Jack, A. S., Matutes, E., Catovsky, D., Hillmen, P. & Houlston, R. S. (2002b). Inherited predisposition to CLL is detectable as subclinical monoclonal B-lymphocyte expansion. *Blood* **100**, 2289–2290.

Rawstron, A. C., de Tute, R., Cullen, M. J., Yuille, M., Kennedy, B., Jack, A. S., Matutes, E., Catovsky, D., Houlston, R. S. & Hillmen, P. (2002c). Sub-Clinical CLL Is found in a High Proportion of "Normal" Relatives from CLL Families: Young Adults Show the Highest Relative Risk. *Blood* **100**, 167.

Risch, N. (1987). Assessing the role of HLA-linked and unlinked determinants of disease. *American Journal of Human Genetics* **40**, 1–14.

Risch, N. & Merikangas, K. (1996). The future of genetic studies of complex human diseases. *Science* **273**, 1516–1517.

Sakai, A., Marti, G. E., Caporaso, N., Pittaluga, S., Touchman, J. W., Fend, F. & Raffeld, M. (2000). Analysis of expressed immunoglobulin heavy chain genes in familial B-CLL. *Blood* **95**, 1413–1419.

Schaffner, C., Stilgenbauer, S., Rappold, G. A., Dohner, H. & Lichter, P. (1999). Somatic ATM mutations indicate a pathogenic role of ATM in B-cell chronic lymphocytic leukaemia. *Blood* **94**, 748–753.

Stankovic, T., Weber, P., Stewart, G., Bedenham, T., Bryd, P. J., Moss, P. A. H. & Taylor, A. M. R. (1999). Inactivation of ataxia telangectasia mutated gene in B-cell chronic lymphocytic leukaemia. *The Lancet* **353**, 26–29.

Summersgill, B., Thornton, P., Atkinson, S., Matutes, E., Shipley, J., Catovsky, D., Houlston, R. S. & Yuille, M. R. (2002). Chromosomal imbalances in familial chronic lymphocytic leukaemia: a comparative genomic hybridisation analysis. *Leukaemia* **16**, 1229–1232.

Swift, M., Reitnauer, P. J., Morrell, D. & Chase, C. L. (1987). Breast and other cancers in families with ataxia-telangiectasia. *New England Journal of Medicine* **316**, 1289–1294.

Taylor, A. M. R., Metcalfe, J. A., Thick, J. & Mak, Y.-F. (1996). Leukaemia and lymphoma in ataxia telangiectasia. *Blood* **87**, 423–428.

Thunberg, U., Tobin, G., Johnson, A., Soderberg, O., Padyukov, L., Hultdin, M., Klareskog, L., Enblad, G., Sundstrom, C., Roos, G. & Rosenquist, R. (2002). Polymorphism in the P2X7 receptor gene and survival in chronic lymphocytic leukaemia. *The Lancet* **360**, 1935–1939.

Wiernik, P. H., Ashwin, M., Hu, X. P., Paietta, E. & Brown, K. (2001). Anticipation in familial chronic lymphocytic leukaemia. *British Journal of Haematology* **113**, 407–414.

Wiley, J. S., Dao-Ung, L. P., Gu, B. J., Sluyter, R., Shemon, A. N., Li, C., Taper, J., Gallo, J. & Manoharan, A. (2002). A loss-of-function polymorphic mutation in the cytolytic P2X7 receptor gene and chronic lymphocytic leukaemia: a molecular study. *The Lancet* **359**, 1114–1119.

Yuille, M. R., Condie, A., Hudson, C. D., Bradshaw, P. S., Stone, E. M., Matutes, E., Catovsky, D. & Houlston, R. S. (2002). ATM mutations are rare in familial chronic lymphocytic leukaemia. *Blood* **100**, 603–609.

Yuille, M. R., Catovsky, D. & Houlston, R. S. (2000b). Pseudoautosomal linkage in chronic lymphocytic leukaemia. *British Journal of Haematology* **109**, 899–900.

Yuille, M. R., Houlston, R. S. & Catovsky, D. (1998). Anticipation in familial chronic lymphocytic leukaemia families. *Leukaemia* **12**, 1696–1698.

Yuille, M. R., Matutes, E., Marossy, A., Hilditch, B., Catovsky, D. & Houlston, R. S. (2000a). Familial chronic lymphocytic leukaemia: a survey and review of published studies. *British Journal of Haematology* **109**, 794–799.

Chapter 2

Cytogenetic and molecular genetic abnormalities in chronic lymphocytic leukaemia

David Oscier and Anne C. Gardiner

Introduction

Early cytogenetic studies in chronic lymphocytic leukaemia (CLL) performed in the 1960s and 1970s failed to detect clonal cytogenetic abnormalities. This inauspicious start to the investigation of genetic abnormalities in CLL was the consequence of the low spontaneous mitotic rate in CLL and the use of the T-cell mitogen phytohaemaglutinin to obtain analysable metaphases. With the discovery of polyclonal B cell mitogens, the first cytogenetic abnormality in CLL, trisomy 12, was discovered in 1980 (Gahrton *et al.* 1980; Hurley *et al.* 1980). Subsequent studies using tetradecanoyl phorbol acetate (TPA) as a mitogen have shown clonal cytogenetic abnormalities in approximately 50% of cases of CLL (Oscier 1994). The most frequent abnormalities are structural abnormalities of chromosome 13q14 and trisomy of chromosome 12 occurring in 10–20% of cases. Abnormalities of chromosomes 6q, 11q, 14q and 17p are each found in less than 5% of cases. In patients with a cytogenetic abnormality, 50% have a single abnormality, 25% have two abnormalities and the remainder have a complex karyotype. Recent studies using either combinations of mitogens including TPA, interleukin 2, tumour necrosis factor alpha and *Staphylococcus aureus* Cowan 1 (Larramendy *et al.* 1998), or CD40 ligand stimulation (Buhmann *et al.* 2002) have revealed clonal cytogenetic abnormalities in 80% of cases. However, mitogens currently employed stimulate normal T cells as well leukaemic B cells; studies that have combined molecular cytogenetic analysis with immunophenotyping of single cells have clearly shown that the normal mitoses in CLL are frequently derived from the normal T cell population (Knuutila *et al.* 1986).

Although cytogenetic analysis has the advantage of providing a global analysis, small deletions and subtle rearrangements cannot be detected. These problems of resolution and the need for metaphases were overcome with the introduction of interphase fluorescent *in situ* hybridisation (FISH). Using centromeric probes specific for individual chromosomes and locus specific probes cloned into yeast artificial chromosome (YAC), P1-derived artificial chromosome, (PAC) or bacterial artificial chromosome (BAC) vectors, the most frequent known abnormalities can be found in 80% of cases of CLL. Comparative genomic hybridisation (CGH) is a further FISH technique, which utilises tumour DNA to enable a global screen for genetic gains, amplifications and losses of tumour DNA. Gains of genetic material on chromosome 4q and 8q have been identified which would not have been predicted from cytogenetic studies (Bentz *et al.* 1995; O'Connor *et al.* 2000). The sensitivity of CGH is greatly enhanced by replacing metaphase chromosomes with micro arrayed DNA fragments as targets (Lichter *et al.* 2000). There are few data on the use of multiplex FISH in CLL. In our experience this technique has been useful in defining the origin of extra chromosomal material in unbalanced rearrangements, and in elucidating complex chromosome rearrangements (Figure 2.1). However, we have not identified additional cryptic abnormalities in patients with trisomy 12, single balanced translocations, or deletions as their sole cytogenetic abnormality (Gardiner *et al.* 2000).

Molecular techniques including Southern analysis and microsatellite analysis to detect loss of heterozygosity have also been employed in CLL. High-resolution allelotyping using a large panel of highly informative microsatellite markers can detect regions of DNA loss not found by routine cytogenetic analysis (Novak *et al.* 2002). Both interphase and metaphase FISH show that the complexity of genetic abnormalities, including the presence of multiple sub-clones, is greater than can be detected from cytogenetic or microsatellite analysis alone (Merup *et al.* 1998b).

Although global studies of gene expression are in their infancy, DNA microarray studies have been performed in CLL and differences in gene expression between CLL and other B cell malignancies and between different cytogenetic subsets of CLL have been identified (Stratowa *et al.* 2001). Proteomic analysis has also shown differences in protein expression between patients with stable or progressive disease (Voss *et al.* 2001), and identified two novel cell surface membrane proteins (Boyd *et al.* 2003).

Chromosome 13q14

Structural abnormalities involving chromosome 13q14 were first noted to be a recurring cytogenetic abnormality in CLL in 1987 (Fitchett *et al.* 1987). Subsequent larger cytogenetic studies have shown that abnormalities of 13q14 are found in approximately 20% of patients, while using more sensitive techniques, the incidence of loss is 30–60%. Two-thirds of patients have a deletion usually at (13)(q14q22) or (13)(q12q14) while the remainder have a translocation involving 13q14. The translocations involve a wide variety of different partner chromosomes, and are frequently complex. FISH analysis of metaphases with 13q14 translocations invariably shows that the translocations are accompanied by genetic loss with variable proximal and distal break points (Figure 2.2) (Gardiner *et al.* 1997).

In contrast to other regions of chromosomal deletion found in CLL, homozygous loss at 13q14 is a frequent finding occurring in 10–20% of cases, strongly suggesting that one or more genes that are important in the pathogenesis of CLL lie within this region.

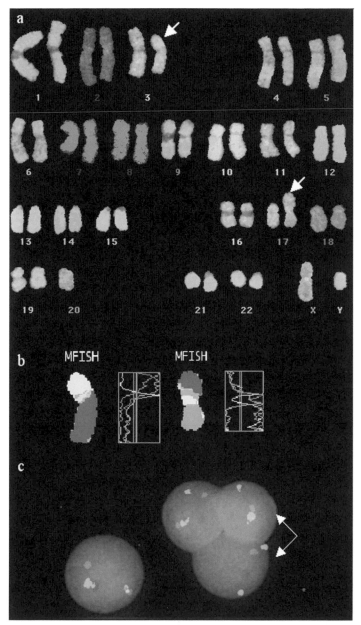

Figure 2.1 (a) M-FISH karyotype from a CLL patient, showing a complex rearrangement involving chromosomes 3, 17 and 20. (b) Abnormal chromosomes 3 and 17 from the karyotype pseudocoloured. Purple indicates chromosome 3, yellow chromosome 17, and pink chromosome 20. (c) Interphase FISH using a probe for chromosome 17 centromere (green), and one for the *p53* gene (red) hybridised to cells from the same patient. Abnormal nuclei (arrowed) show only one p53 signal.

(The editors regret that it has not been possible to print this figure as a colour illustration. A colour version is available from the first author by e-mail).

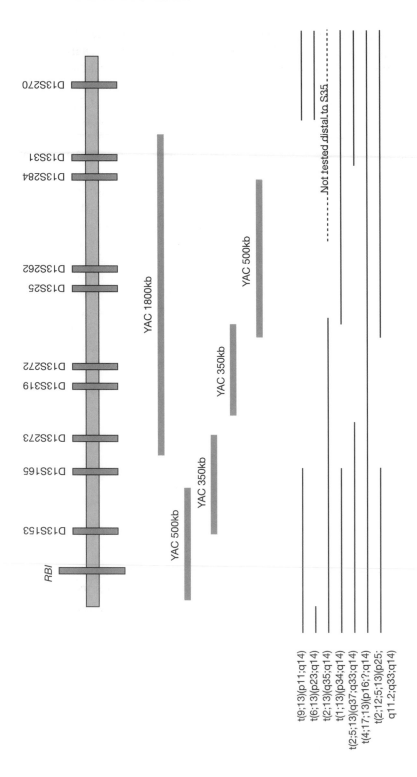

Figure 2.2 Chromosome 13q14 showing the positions of a series of YACs used to determine the breakpoints of a series of seven patients with translocations involving 13q14 shown in the lower section of the figure.

Several groups constructed detailed physical maps of 13q14 and have performed deletion mapping using either FISH, Southern or microsatellite analysis. Several overlapping regions of minimal genetic loss have been identified and these are shown in Figure 2.3. A 10 kilobase (kb) region of minimal loss close to D13S319 encompasses exons of two separate transcripts termed *LEU1* and *LEU2*, neither of which encode a protein product (Liu *et al.* 1997). The *RFP2* gene is located 50 kb centromeric of the minimally deleted region on chromosome 13 and encodes a 407 amino acid ring-finger protein which shares homology with several transcription factors including *BRCA2* (Kapanadze *et al.* 1998). Sequence analysis of the corresponding mouse genomic region has revealed strong identity between the human and mouse *LEU2* and *RFP2* genes (Kapanadze *et al.* 2000). Although *LEU1, LEU2 and RFP2* may be considered as strong candidate genes, no mutations have been found in these genes, their promotor regions, or in other genes in the deleted region. Nor is there evidence for CpG island methylation of these genes on the remaining allele in patients with heterozygous loss in this region (Migliazza *et al.* 2001; Mertens *et al.* 2002; Van Everdink *et al.* 3003). Recently, deletion and reduced expression of two non coding micro-RNA genes, miR15 and miR16, which lie within the LEU2 gene in the minimally deleted region has been detected in the majority of patients with 13q loss (Calin *et al.* 2002). The mechanism whereby hetero- or homozygous loss of these genes influences the pathogenesis of CLL remains unclear.

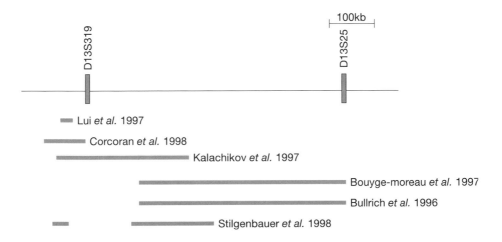

Figure 2.3 Minimal regions of 13q14 loss, indicated by solid lines, found in six studies.

Table 2.1 Incidence of trisomy 12 in CLL

Study	Number of patients	+12 determined by cytogenetics (%)	+12 determined by interphase FISH (%)
Perez-Losada *et al.* (1991)	13	0	15
Anastasi *et al.* (1992)	40	18	30
Que *et al.* (1993)	118	9	14
Escudier *et al.* (1993)	117	13	35
Dohner *et al.* (1993)	42	10	14
Criel *et al.* (1997)	111	12	14
Oscier *et al.* (2002)	205	29	30

Trisomy 12

Trisomy 12 is by far the most frequent numerical chromosome abnormality in CLL. Using restriction fragment length polymorphism studies, the additional chromosome 12 has been shown to derive from duplication of one chromosome 12 homologue with retention of the other homologue, rather than from triplication of a single homologue (Einhorn *et al.* 1989). The incidence of trisomy 12, in studies which have used both cytogenetic and interphase FISH analysis is shown in Table 2.1. The wide variation in incidence may partly reflect the extent to which studies include patients with atypical lymphocyte morphology, which as discussed later, is strongly associated with trisomy 12.

The genetic consequence of trisomy 12 is unknown. Clues to the identity of the key gene or genes on chromosome 12 may come from the investigation of rare cases with translocations, duplications, or genomic amplifications involving chromosome 12. Two cases in which CLL had transformed to diffuse large-cell lymphoma were shown to have translocations involving 12p13 and 12q13 respectively. In the first case there was disruption of the Cyclin D2 promoter (Qian *et al.* 1999). In the second, the translocation occurred within the *HMGI-C* gene, which encodes a high mobility group protein known to be over expressed in a variety of malignancies (Santulli *et al.* 2000). Dysregulation of the chondroitin 4-0-Sulfotransferase 1 gene has been reported in a single case of CLL with t(12;14) (q23; q32) (Schmidt *et al.* 2000). In a study of duplications resulting in partial trisomy 12 in patients with low grade B cell malignancies, a duplicated region between q13 and q22 was identified in patients with CLL (Dierlamm *et al.* 1997). This region includes the *MDM2* gene; the possible significance of this gene in CLL is discussed below.

Chromosome 11q

Using a panel of YAC probes spanning 11q14–q23 Stilgenbauer *et al.* (1996) investigated 38 patients with CLL who had cytogenetic deletions of chromosome 11q.

A commonly deleted region of between 2 and 3 Mb at 11q22.3–q23.1 was identified. In two additional cases with 11q translocations, the translocation break points were localised to the commonly deleted region. In a subsequent larger interphase FISH study, 43 of 214 cases were found to have heterozygous loss of a YAC within the minimally deleted region (Dohner *et al.* 1997). This high incidence of loss contrasts with previous cytogenetic studies in which 11q22–23 abnormalities were found in less than 5% of cases. Trinucleotide repeat sequences have been found close to the chromosome breakpoints in cases with deletion of 11q, and these may be responsible for increased chromosome fragility (Auer *et al.* 2001). The minimally deleted region contains several candidate tumour suppresser genes including *RDX* which has homology to the neurofibromatosis type 2 gene (*NF2 71*), *PPP2RIB* a phosphatase which is mutated in sporadic cases of lung and colon cancer and *ATM* which is mutated in Ataxia Telangectasia. Mutation of the *PPP2RIB* gene or loss of phosphatase activity, have not been found in cases of CLL with deletion of one copy of the *PPP2RIB* gene (Schaffner *et al.* 2000).

The *ATM* gene encodes a 350kd protein, which plays a crucial role in recognising and orchestrating the cellular response to double stranded DNA breaks caused by irradiation. *ATM* mutations in CLL occur throughout the coding region and include both missense mutations and truncating mutations or deletions. Loss of the remaining allele is unusual (Pettitt *et al.* 2001; Stankovic *et al.* 2002). These features are in contrast to those seen in mantle cell lymphoma and T prolymphocytic leukaemia in which predominantly missense mutations are clustered within the catalytic PI-3Kinase domain and the normal allele is lost (Camacho *et al.* 2002). Abnormalities of *ATM* may be detected by mutational analysis of the *ATM* gene, measurement of ATM protein levels by Western blotting, or by functional assays which show failure to upregulate *ATM*-dependent proteins following exposure of CLL cells to gamma irradiation (Starostik *et al.* 1998; Bullrich *et al.* 1999; Stankovic *et al.* 1999, 2004). There is a close but not absolute correlation between these assays. *ATM* mutations are predominantly found in patients with unmutated IgVH genes and are detected in 10–15% of these cases. It is still unclear what percentage of patients with 11q deletions and loss of a single copy of the *ATM* gene detected by FISH, have an abnormality of the *ATM* gene on the remaining homologue and a pathogenetic role for other genes on 11q has not been excluded (Schaffner *et al.* 1999; Zhu *et al.* 1999). One candidate is the *H2AX* gene, which plays a role in the repair of double stranded DNA breaks. This gene is located 11 Mb telomeric to *ATM*, and mice deficient in both *H2AX* and *p53* develop lymphoid tumours (Celeste *et al.* 2003; Bassing *et al.* 2003).

Chromosome 17p

Structural abnormalities involving chromosome 17p include translocations, deletions and isochromosome of 17q, and are found in 5% of patients with CLL. In a recent study using FISH, 10 out of 14 cases with 17p translocations were shown to have dicentric rearrangements, raising the possibility that telomere shortening may have preceded the chromosomal event (Callet-Bauchu *et al.* 1999). These abnormalities usually result in loss of the *p53* gene located at 17p13 and are frequently accompanied by mutation of the *p53* gene on the other allele.

The *p53* gene encodes a tetrameric DNA binding protein, which is upregulated in response to a variety of cellular stress signals including irradiation and chemotherapeutic agents. p53 induces the expression of numerous genes such as *p21* involved in cell cycle arrest, *BAX*, which is pro-apoptotic, and MDM2 which acts as a negative regulator and promotes p53 degradation. Cells which lack wild-type p53 protein are resistant to being killed by irradiation or drugs such as alkylating agents and are susceptible to further DNA damage and chromosome abnormalities induced by these agents.

p53 gene mutations are usually missense mutations affecting hot spots in exons 4 to 8, and result in the expression of a mutant protein which is unable to bind DNA and which may interfere with the function of residual wild-type protein. *p53* abnormalities may be detected using a variety of techniques including single strand confirmation polymorphism analysis, genomic sequencing, FISH analysis and increased p53 protein expression using immunocytochemistry or flow cytometry. However, techniques which rely on protein expression miss both frameshift and nonsense mutations which lack a protein product. Lin *et al.* (2002) have developed a functional assay which detects both *p53* and *ATM* mutations. CLL cells are irradiated in vitro and p53 and p21 expression are measured using flow cytometry. Patients with a missense *p53* mutation express p53 but not p21 whereas those with an *ATM* mutation fail to express either protein. It is possible that other defects in the p53 pathway such as overexpression of MDM2 could be detected by this assay. Over expression of MDM2 mRNA and/or protein in CLL has been shown in several studies (Bueso-Ramos *et al.* 1993, Huang *et al.* 1994, Watanabe *et al.* 1994). However, neither the mechanism of over expression nor the clinical significance is understood.

P53 mutation or deletion is reported in 7–30% of patients with CLL (Table 2.2). The varying incidence is partly technical but largely reflects patient selection, as mutations are most commonly found in cases with advanced disease and unmutated IgVH genes.

Immunoglobulin gene translocations

Chromosomal translocations involving the immunoglobulin loci are both frequent and critical to the pathogenesis of many chronic lymphoproliferative disorders, but are rare in CLL.

The incidence of rearrangement involving the *BCL2* locus is shown in Table 2.4. Initial studies noted a high incidence of translocation involving the immunoglobulin light chain loci, but in our own series (Gardiner *et al.* 2003) 14 of 17 cases had t(14:18)(q32q21) translocations. The breakpoints within the *BCL2* locus are variable,

Table 2.2 p53 mutation or deletion in chronic lymphocytic leukaemia

Study	Number of patients	Method	Mutation or Loss (%)
Gaidano *et al.* (1991)	40	SSCP/PCR	15
Fenaux *et al.* (1992)	39	SSCP/PCR	10
El Rouby *et al.* (1993)	53	SSCP/PCR	15
Dohner *et al.* (1995)	16	FISH	25
Lens *et al.* (1997)	32	"17p LOH,Immuno-" "cytochemistry, p53 " sequence.	30
Cordone *et al.* (1998)	181	"Immunocytochemistry," p53 sequence.	15
Dohner *et al.* (2000)	325	FISH	7
Oscier *et al.* (2002)	202	Karyotype	6
	90	FISH	6
	155	FLOW	4.5

but frequently involve the 5′ variable cluster region in those cases with immunoglobulin light chain translocations and the major breakpoint cluster in cases which translocate to the immunoglobulin heavy chain. Many cases of immunoglobulin gene/*BCL2* rearrangements are accompanied by trisomy 12 and the *BCL2* rearrangement may be the primary or secondary cytogenetic abnormality. It is intriguing that cases in which the *BCL2* translocation is a primary event have mutated IgVH genes whereas secondary *BCL2* translocations are associated with unmutated IgVH genes.

Translocations involving the immunoglobulin heavy chain locus on chromosome 14q32 and the *BCL3* gene on 19q13 are found in less than 0.5% of patients. The breakpoints in the immunoglobulin heavy chain gene are usually in the switch region upstream of C-alpha 1 or C-alpha 2 (Ohno *et al.* 1993). The *BCL3* breakpoints are variable but all result in over expression of the BCL3 protein, which is an I-kappa-B-like protein. Most cases have complex cytogenetic abnormalities including trisomy 12 (Michaux *et al.* 1997, McKeithan *et al.* 1997).

The t(2;14) (p13;q32) is a rare recurring translocation in B cell malignancies and has been studied molecularly in four clinically aggressive cases of CLL. A zinc finger gene (*BCL 11A*) is juxtaposed to the immunoglobulin heavy chain locus. *BCL 11A* interacts with *BCL6,* both of which are transcriptional repressors (Satterwhite *et al.* 2001).

The existence of the t(11:14) in CLL is controversial. In almost all reported cases, lymphocyte morphology is atypical and the immunophenotype is more consistent with mantle cell lymphoma than CLL. Gene expression profiling has shown that indolent cases with a t(11;14) lymphocytosis and no lymphadenopathy have a profile typical of mantle cell lymphoma rather than CLL (Oscier *et al.* 2002).

Chromosome 6q

Structural abnormalities of chromosome 6 predominantly involve the long arm and comprise deletions affecting bands q21, q23, q25-27, or more rarely translocations which also involve a variety of breakpoints.

The incidence of chromosome 6q deletions was 6% in a cytogenetic analysis of 662 cases and 7% in a FISH analysis of 285 patients using a YAC probe mapping to band 6q21 (Stilgenbauer *et al.* 1999). Merup *et al.* (1998a) observed a minimally deleted region between the microsatellite markers D6S283 and D6S270, which includes the candidate gene *TLX*, a member of the nuclear steroid receptor superfamily.

Telomere length and telomerase activity

Telomeres are essential for both the function and stability of normal chromosomes. Repeated cell division results in telomere shortening and in most somatic cells, which are unable to activate telomerase, eventually leads to cell senescence or apoptosis. Normal B cells undergo age-dependent telomere shortening but can upregulate telomerase in response to antigenic stimulation. Telomere elongation occurs in germinal centre B cells accounting for the longer telomeres of $CD27^+$ memory B cells compared with $CD27^-$ naive B cells (Martens *et al.* 2002). Several studies have documented increased telomerase activity and reduced telomere length in advanced CLL compared to patients with stage A disease (Counter *et al.* 1995; Bechter *et al.* 1998) and in unmutated compared with mutated cases (Hultdin *et al.* 2003; Damle *et al.* 2003). Telomere length is uniformly short in unmutated cases, possibly reflecting compensatory telomerase activity. However, there is greater heterogeneity in telomere length in mutated cases and a moderate association between long telomeres and high IgVH gene mutational load, consistent with greater telomere elongation and mutational activity in germinal centre cells undergoing multiple rounds of cell division. The longer telomeres of mutated cases, may reflect the indolent nature of this subset in which proliferative activity is low. Alternatively, the final transforming event in mutated cases may occur in a cell with longer telomeres than the target cell in the unmutated subset. The latter hypothesis is supported by the analysis of serial samples from both subsets showing a comparable rate of decrease in telomere length (Damle *et al.* 2003).

Timing and evolution of genetic abnormalities in CLL

Clues to the nature of the genetic event(s) that may initiate leukaemogenesis come from a variety of sources. Patients with early CLL and healthy individuals with a clonal lymphocytosis, detected by using sensitive flow cytometric assays designed to detect minimal residual disease, frequently have deletions of 13q14 as the sole cytogenetic abnormality, suggesting that genetic loss in this region is an early event. Croce (2003) has developed a mouse model of CLL by introducing a *TCL1* transgene into B cells. At 12 months the transgenic mice develop a clonal CD5 positive lymphocytosis and interestingly many of these mice acquire deletions of the miR15 and miR16 genes on the murine homologue of human chromosome 13q.

Further progress in defining initiating events should come from the current detailed analysis of patients with familial CLL (Houlston *et al.* 2002). Linkage studies have identified several loci, including 13q14, which may harbour a 'CLL gene' but key genes are still awaiting discovery. Rarely, patients with a somatic mutation of the *ATM* gene also carry a germline *ATM* mutation, raising the possibility that germline *ATM* mutations are an important cause of familial CLL. However, a recent linkage analysis of 28 families did not support this hypothesis (Bevan *et al.* 1999). Provocative data from Stankovic *et al.* (2002) identified two patients with CLL and somatic *ATM* mutations in which the *ATM* mutations were also found in other haemopoietic lineages, suggesting that the mutation may be acquired early in haematopoiesis before both B-cell commitment and to the onset of leukaemogenesis.

In most human tumours, genetic abnormalities accumulate during the course of the disease and contribute to disease progression and drug resistance. Sequential cytogenetic and interphase FISH studies have demonstrated clonal evolution in 10–20% of cases (Juliusson *et al.* 1988; Oscier 1994) and confirmed that deletions of chromosome 6q, 11q and 17p are the most frequent secondary abnormalities (Fegan *et al.* 1995; Finn *et al.* 1998; Cuneo *et al.* 2002). Stilgenbauer (2003a) studied four patients who developed biallelic p53 abnormalities during the course of their disease. Serial analysis showed that these abnormalities were either only detectable after treatment or the percentage of cells with p53 abnormalities increased after therapy, implying that treatment was effective against the wild-type p53 clone and selected for the drug resistant p53 mutant clone.

Trisomy 12 is almost invariably a primary cytogenetic abnormality in CLL, but interphase FISH has shown that only part of the leukaemic clone carries the additional copy of chromosome 12 (Garcia-Marco *et al.* 1994).

In patients with CLL who develop a diffuse large-cell lymphoma (Richter syndrome) the new clone may either be derived from the CLL clone or be unrelated. In those cases in which the large cell lymphoma is clonally related to CLL, studies on small numbers of patients have not shown a consistent transforming event (Matolcsy *et al.* 1994).

The clinical significance of genetic abnormalities in CLL

Data from the first and second International Working Party on Chromosomes in CLL, which included many patients with prolonged follow-up, found the median survival of patients with a normal karyotype to be 15 years compared with 7.7 years for patients with a clonal abnormality. Patients with complex karyotypic abnormalities had a poorer survival time than patients with either a normal karyotype or a single abnormality. When patients with single abnormalities only were studied, those with trisomy 12 had a poorer prognosis than patients with abnormalities of chromosome 13, or those with a normal karyotype (Juliusson *et al.* 1990, 1991).

The results of the most comprehensive univariate analysis of the prognostic significance of genetic abnormalities in 325 cases of CLL analysed by interphase FISH for deletions of 6q, 11q, 13q and 17p, trisomies of 3q, 8q and 12q and translocations involving 14q32 are shown in Table 2.3 (Dohner *et al.* 2000).

However, interpretation of the clinical significance of cytogenetic abnormalities is complicated by their association with other clinical and laboratory features which also have prognostic significance in univariate analysis (Table 2.4).

Table 2.3 Incidence and clinical significance of genetic abnormalities in chronic lymphocytic leukaemia

Genetic abnormality	Incidence (%)	Median survival (months)	Median treatment-free survival (months)
del 13q	55	133*	92
del 11q	18	79	13
trisomy 12q	16	114	33
del 17p	7	32	9
No abnormality	18	111	49

* For patients with del 13q as the sole genetic abnormality. From Dohner *et al.* (2000)

Table 2.4 Genetic abnormality and clinical correlation in CLL

Genetic abnormality	Clinical correlation
del13q	"typical morphology," "mutated VH genes," stable disease.
del6q	extensive lymphadenopathy
+12	"atypical morphology," ? progressive disease.
del 11q23	"bulky lymphadenopathy," "progressive disease," early relapse post autograft.
p53 loss or mutation	"atypical morphology," advanced disease drug resistance.

More recently, two large studies have performed multivariate analyses with included IgVH gene mutational status and CD38 expression. Both studies confirmed the prognostic significance of IgVH gene mutations and found that deletion of chromosome 11q and loss of the *p53* gene occur more frequently in unmutated cases. Both studies also showed that *p53* loss or mutation was an independent poor prognostic factor in all cases and in those with Binet stage A disease (Figure 2.4) (Oscier *et al.* 2002; Krober *et al.* 2002). Chromosome 11q deletion was not an independent poor risk factor in one of the studies (Oscier *et al.* 2002), and was only significant when the cut off for IgVH gene homology to the germline was taken as 98% rather than 97% in the other.

Many, but not all, previous studies had shown an association between *p53* loss and/or mutation with advanced clinical stage, an increase in circulating prolymphocytes, rapid disease progression, a poor response to therapy with alkylating agents and purine analogues and short survival (El Rouby *et al.* 1993; Wattel *et al.* 1994; Dohner *et al.* 1995; Lens *et al.* 1997; Barnabas *et al.* 2001). However, patients with *p53* mutations may still be responsive to high-dose methylprednisolone and to alemtuzumab (Stilgenbauer *et al.* 2003b; Thornton *et al.* 2003).

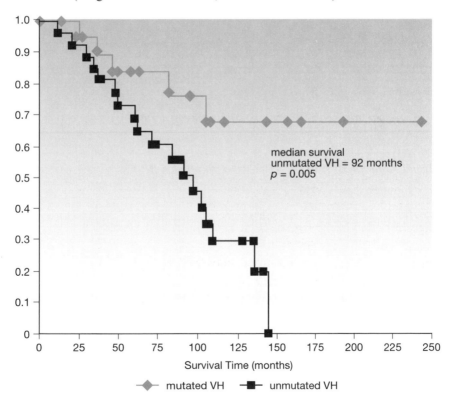

Figure 2.4 Survival curve comparing trisomy 12 patients with mutated and unmutated immunoglobulin V genes.

The lack of a clear association between 11q deletion and poor outcome was surprising in view of the results of previous studies. In 1997, Dohner *et al.* and Neilson *et al.* reported that deletion of 11q22–q23 was associated with rapid disease progression and poor survival. In addition, patients with 11q deletions presented at a younger age and with more advanced disease, particularly with bulky lymphadenopathy. Of particular interest was the finding that the poor survival of patients with 11q deletions was confined to patients younger than 55 years of age. The explanation for the impact of age on survival is unclear because in general, younger patients with CLL do not have a more aggressive disease than elderly patients. In the CLL3 trial of the German CLL Study Group, deletion of 11q was associated with molecular evidence of persistent disease following autologous stem cell transplantation in 38% of cases compared with 6% of cases without an 11q deletion (Stilgenbauer *et al.* 2000). Larger studies, which include data on *ATM* mutations, are required to determine the importance of genetic loss at 11q in CLL.

Although there is a consensus that isolated deletion of 13q is associated with a favourable prognosis, the influence of trisomy 12 on survival remains controversial. Trisomy 12 is closely associated with atypical lymphocyte morphology. Criel *et al.* (1997) found trisomy 12 to be an adverse prognostic factor only in patients with typical lymphocyte morphology. In a multivariate analysis, which included both trisomy 12 and lymphocyte morphology, only lymphocyte morphology retained prognostic significance (Oscier *et al.* 1997). Our own data demonstrated a median survival of 95 months for patients with trisomy 12 and unmutated VH genes, whereas the median survival has not been reached for patients with VH gene mutations (p = 0.005) (Figure 2.5) Gardiner *et al.* 2000).

Patients with chromosome 6q deletions have a higher white cell count and more extensive lymphadenopathy than patients without 6q deletions but there is no impact on either treatment-free or overall survival (Stilgenbauer *et al.* 1999).

Until recently, cytogenetic data have been collected in large national CLL trials such as the MRC CLL4 trial and the German CLL trials, but the data have not influenced patient management. However, a current European study stratifies previously untreated Binet stage A patients based on IgVH gene status, serum thymidine kinase, lymphocyte doubling time and *p53* and 11q loss. Patients with two or more poor risk factors are randomised to early or delayed treatment.

Conclusion

The combination of cytogenetic analysis, interphase FISH and CGH has identified genetic abnormalities in over 80% of cases of CLL. The incidence of abnormalities is highest in patients with advanced disease whereas deletion of chromosome 13q14 is the only consistent abnormality in patients with a stable mild lymphocytosis.

Deletions of chromosome 17p and 11q occur mainly in patients with unmutated IgVH genes and are adverse prognostic factors. Deletions of chromosome 13q and

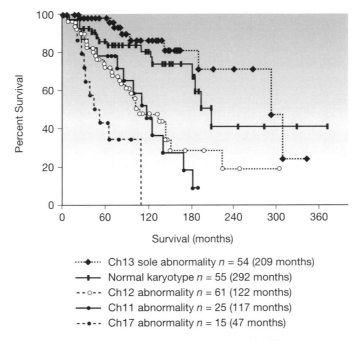

 Ch13 sole abnormality *n* = 54 (209 months)
Normal karyotype *n* = 55 (292 months)
Ch12 abnormality *n* = 61 (122 months)
Ch11 abnormality *n* = 25 (117 months)
Ch17 abnormality *n* = 15 (47 months)

Figure 2.5 Impact of genetic abnormalities on survival in CLL.

trisomy 12 do not have independent prognostic significance and the apparently poorer survival of patients with trisomy 12 largely reflects the association between trisomy 12 and unmutated VH genes.

It can be expected that a fuller understanding of the molecular consequences of 13q deletions will provide greater insight into the pathogenesis of early CLL, while the key therapeutic issue in this disease is the development of new strategies to treat patients with mutations of the *ATM / p53* pathway.

References

Anastasi J., LeBeau, M. M., Vardiman, J. W., Fernald, A. A., Larson, R. A. & Rowley, J. D. (1992). Detection of trisomy 12 in chronic lymphocytic leukemia by fluorescence in situ hybridization to interphase cells: a simple and sensitive method. *Blood* **79**, 1796–1801.

Auer, R. L., Jones, C., Mullenbach, R. A., Syndercombe-Court, D., Milligan, D. W., Fegan C. & Cotter, F. E. (2001). Role for CCG-trinucleotide repeats in the pathogenesis of chronic lymphocytic leukemia. *Blood* **97**, 509–515.

Barnabas, N., Shurafa, M., Van Dyke, D. L., Wolman, S.R., Clark, D. & Worsham, M. J. (2001). Significance of p53 mutations in patients with chronic lymphocytic leukaemia. *Cancer* **91**, 285–293.

Bassing, C. H., Suh, H., Ferguson, D. O., Chua, K. F., Manis, J., Eckersdorff, M., Gleason M., Bronson, R., Lee, C. & Alt. F. W. (2003). Histone H2AX: a dosage-dependent suppressor of oncogenic translocations and tumours. *Cell* **114**, 359–370.

Bechter, O. E., Eisterer, W. P. G., Hilbe, W., Kuhr, T. & Thaler, J. (1998). Telomere length and telomerase activity predict survival in patients with B cell chronic lymphocytic leukemia. *Cancer Research* **21**, 4918–4922.

Bentz, M., Huck, K., du Manoir, S., Joos, S., Werner, C. A., Fischer, K., Dohner, H. & Lichter, P. (1995). Comparative genomic hybridization in chronic B-cell leukemias shows a high incidence of chromosomal gains and losses. *Blood* **85**, 3610–3618.

Bevan, S., Catovsky, D., Marossy, A., Matutes, E., Popat, S., Antonovic, P., Bell, A., Berrebi Gaminara, E. J., Quabeck, K. and 9 others (1999). Linkage analysis for *ATM* in familial B cell chronic lymphocytic leukaemia. *Leukemia* **13**, 1497–1500.

Bueso-Ramos, C. E., Yang, Y., deLeon, E., McCown, P., Stass, S. A. & Albitar, M. (1993). The human MDM-2 oncogene is overexpressed in leukemias. *Blood* **82**, 2617–2623.

Bouyge-Moreau, I., Rondeau, G., Avet-Loiseau, H., Andre, M. T., Bezieau, S., Cherel, M. Saleun, S., Cadoret, E., Shaikh, T., de Angelis, M. M. and 4 others (1997). Construction of a 780-kb PAC., BAC., and cosmid contig encompassing the minimal critical deletion involved in B cell chronic lymphocytic leukemia at 13q14.3. *Genomics* **46**, 183–190.

Boyd, R. S., Adams, P. J., Patel, S., Loader, J. A., Redpath, N. T., Poyser, H. R., Fletcher, G. C., Burgess, N. A., Stamps, A. C., Hudson, L. and 8 others (2003). Proteomic analysis of the cell-surface membrane in chronic lymphocytic leukaemia: identification of two novel proteins., BCNP1 and MIG2B. *Leukemia* **17**, 1605–1612

Buhmann, R., Kurzeder, C., Rehklau, J., Westhaus, D., Bursch, S., Hiddemann, W., Haferlach, T., Hallek, M. & Schoch, C. (2002). CD40L stimulation enhances the ability of conventional metaphase cytogenetics to detect chromosome aberrations in B-cell chronic lymphocytic leukaemia cells. *British Journal of Haematology* **118**, 968–975.

Bullrich, F., Veronese M. L., Kitada, S., Jurlander, J., Caliguiri, M. A., Reed, J. C. & Croce, C. M. (1996). Minimal region of loss at 13q14 in B-cell chronic lymphocytic leukemia. *Blood* **88**, 3109–3115.

Bullrich, F., Rasio, D., Kitada, S., Starostik, P., Kipps, T., Keating, M., Albitar, M., Reed, J. C. & Croce, C. M. (1999). *ATM* mutations in B-cell chronic lymphocytic leukemia *Cancer Research* **59**, 24–27.

Calin, G.A., Dumitru, C. D., Shimizu, M., Bichi, R., Zupo, S., Noch, E., Aldler, H., Rattan, S., Keating, M., Rai, K., Rassenti, L., Kipps, T., Negrini, M., Bullrich, F. & Croce, C. M. (2002). Frequent deletions and down-regulation of micro-RNA genes miR15 and miR16 at 13q14 in chronic lymphocytic leukaemia. *Proceedings of the National Academy of Sciences of the United States of America* **99**, 15,524–15,529.

Callet-Bauchu, E., Salles, G., Gazzo, S., Poncet, C., Morel, D., Pages, J., Coiffier, B Coeur, P. & Felman, P. (1999). Translocations involving the short arm of chromosome 17 in chronic B–lymphoid disorders: frequent occurrence of dicentric rearrangements and possible association with adverse outcome. *Leukemia* **13**, 460–468.

Camacho, E., Hernandez, L., Herrnandez, S., Tort, F., Bellosillo, B., Bea, S., Bosch, F., Montserrat, E., Cardesa, A., Fernandez, P. L. & Campo, E. (2002). ATM gene inactivation in mantle cell lymphoma mainly occurs by truncating mutations and missense mutations involving the phosphatidylinositol-3 kinase domain and is associated with increasing numbers of chromosomal imbalances. *Blood* **99**, 238–244.

Celeste, A., Difilippantonio, S., Difilipantonio, M. J., Fernandez-Capetillo, O., Pilch, D. R., Sedelnikova, O. A., Eckhaus, M., Ried, T., Bonner, W. M. & Nussenweig, A. (2003). H2AX haploinsufficiency modifies genomic stability and tumour susceptibility. *Cell* **114**, 371–383.

Corcoran, M. M., Rasool, O., Liu, Y., Iyengar, A., Grander, D., Ibbotson, R. E., Merup, M., Wu, S., Brodyansky, V., Gardiner, A. C. and 9 others (1998). Detailed molecular delineation of 13q14.3 loss in B-cell chronic lymphocytic leukemia. *Blood* **91**, 1–10.

Cordone, I., Masi, S., Mauro, F. R., Soddu, S., Morsilli, O., Valentini, T., Vegna, M. L., Guglielmi C., Mancini F., Giuliacci S. and 3 others (1998). p53xpression in B-cell chronic lymphocytic leukemia: A marker of disease progression and poor prognosis. *Blood* **91**, 4342–4349.

Counter, C. M., Gupta, J., Harley, C. B., Leber, B. & Bacchetti, S. (1995). Telomerase activity in normal leukocytes and in hematologic malignancies. *Blood* **85**, 2315–2320.

Criel, A., Verhoef, G., Vlietinck, R., Mecucci, C., Billiet, J., Michaux, L., Meeus, P., Louwagie, A., Can Orshoven, A., Van Hoof, A. and 3 others (1997). Further characterization of morphologically defined typical and atypical CLL: a clinical, immunophenotypic, cytogenetic and prognostic study on 390 cases. *British Journal of Haematology* **97**, 383–391.

Croce, C. M. (2003). Animal models in CLL. *Leukemia and Lymphoma* **44** (Suppl. 2) S2.

Cuneo, A., Bigoni, R., Rigolin, G. M., Boberti, M. G., Bardi, A., Cavazzini, F.,Milani, R., Minotto, C., Della Porta, M., Agostini, P. and 3 others (2002). Late appearance of the 11q22.3–23.1 deletion involving the ATM locus in B cell chronic lymphocytic leukaemia and related disorders. *Haematologica* **87**, 44–51.

Damle, R. N., Batliwalla, F. M., Albesionao, E., Valetto, A., Allen, S. L., Schulman, P., Vinciguerra V., Rai, K., Ferrarini, M., Gregersen, P. K. & Chiorazzi, N. (2000). Telomere length analysis suggests distinct replicative histories of B-CLL subgroups. *Blood* **96**(Suppl.), 836a.

Dierlamm, J., Wlodarska I., Michaux L., Vermeesch, J. R., Meeus, P., Stul M., Verhoef G., Thomas J., Delannoy A., Louwagie A. and 3 others (1997). FISH identifies different types of duplications in 12q13-15 as the commonly involved segment in B-cell lymphoproliferative malignancies characterized by partial trisomy 12 *Genes, Chromosomes and Cancer* **20**, 155–166.

Dohner, H., Pohl, S., Bulgay-Morschel, M., Stilgenbauer, S., Bentz, M. & Lichter, P. (1993). Trisomy 12 in chronic lymphoid leukemias – a metaphase and interphase cytogenetic analysis. *Leukemia* **7**, 516–520.

Dohner, H., Fischer, K., Bentz, M., Hansen, K., Benner, A., Cabot, G., Diehl, D., Schlenk, R., Coy, J., Stilgenbauer, S. and 5 others (1995). p53 gene deletion predicts for poor survival and non-response to therapy with purine analogs in chronic B-cell leukemias. *Blood* **85**, 1580–1589.

Dohner, H., Stilgenbauer, S., James, M., Benner, A., Weilguni, T., Bentz, M., Fischer, K Hunstein, W. & Lichter, P. (1997). 11q deletions identify a new subset of B-cell chronic lymphocytic leukemia characterized by extensive nodal involvement and inferior prognosis. *Blood* **89**, 2516–2522.

Dohner, H., Stilgenbauer, S., Benner, A., Leupolt, E., Krober, A., Bullinger, L., Dohner, K., Bentz, M. & Lichter, P. (2000). Genomic aberrations and survival in chronic lymphocytic leukemia. *New England Journal of Medicine* **343**, 1910–1916.

Drandi, D., Lee, C., Dal Cin, P. & Gribben, J. (2003). Array-based comparative genomic hybridisation identifies deletion at 14q32 as a new prognostic marker in chronic lymphocytic leukaemia *Blood* **102**(Suppl.), 186a

Einhorn, S., Burvall, K., Juliusson, G., Gahrton, G. & Meeker, T. (1989). Molecular analyses of chromosome 12 in chronic lymphocytic leukemia. *Leukemia* **3**, 871–874.

El Rouby, S., Thomas, A., Costin, D., Rosenberg, C. R., Potmesil, M., Silber, R. & Newcomb, E. (1993). p53 gene mutation in B-cell chronic lymphocytic leukemia is associated with drug resistance and is independent of MDR1/MDR3 gene expression. *Blood* **82**, 3452–3459.

Escudier, S. M., Pereira-Leahy, J. M., Drach, J. W., Weier, H. U., Goodacre, A. M., Cork, M. A., Trujillo, J. M., Keating, M. J. & Andreeff, M. (1993). Fluorescent in situ hybridization and cytogenetic studies of trisomy 12 in chronic lymphocytic leukemia. *Blood* **81**, 1702–2707.

Fegan, C., Robinson, H., Thompson, P., Whittaker, J. A. & White, D. (1995). Karyotypic evolution in CLL: identification of a new sub-group of patients with deletions of 11q and advanced or progressive disease. *Leukemia* **9**, 2003–2008.

Fenaux, P., Preudhomme, C., Lai, J. L., Quiquandon, I., Jonveaux, P. Vanrumbeke, M., Sartiaux, C., Morel, P., Loucheux-Lefebvre, M. H., Bauters, F. and 2 others (1992). Mutations of the p53 gene in B-cell chronic lymphocytic leukemia: a report on 39 cases with cytogenetic analysis. *Leukemia* **6**, 246–250.

Finn, W. G., Kay, N. E., Kroft, S. H., Church, S. & Peterson, L. C. (1998). Secondary abnormalities of chromosome 6q in B-cell chronic lymphocytic leukemia: A sequential study of karyotypic instability in 51 patients. *American Journal of Haematology* **59**, 223–229.

Fitchett, M., Griffiths, M. J., Oscier, D. G., Johnson, S. & Seabright, M. (1987). Chromosome abnormalities involving band 13q14 in hematologic malignancies. *Cancer Genetics and Cytogenetics* **24**, 143–150.

Gahrton, G., Robert, K. H., Friberg, K., Zech, L. & Bird, A. G. (1980). Extra chromosome 12 in chronic lymphocytic leukemia. *The Lancet* **i**, 146–147.

Gaidano, G., Ballerini, P., Gong, J. Z., Inghirami, G., Neri, A., Newcomb, E. W., Macgrath, I. T., Knowles, D. M. & Dalla Favera, R. (1991). p53 mutations in human lymphoid malignancies: Association with Burkitt lymphoma and chronic lymphocytic leukemia. *Proceedings of the National Academy of Sciences of the United States of America* **88**, 5413–5417.

Garcia-Marco, J., Matutes, E., Morilla, R., Ellis, J., Oscier, D., Fantes, J., Catovsky, D. & Price, C. M. (1994). Trisomy 12 in B-cell chronic lymphocytic leukaemia: assessment of lineage restriction by simultaneous analysis of immunophenotype and genotype in interphase cells by fluorescence *in situ* hybridization. *British Journal of Haematology* **87**, 44–50.

Gardiner, A. C., Corcoran, M. M. & Oscier, D. G. (1997). Cytogenetic., fluorescence in situ hybridisation., and clinical evaluation of translocations with concomitant deletion at 13q14 in chronic lymphocytic leukaemia. *Genes, Chromosomes and Cancer* **20**, 73–81.

Gardiner, A. C., Mould, S. J., Glide, S., Davis, Z. A., Orchard, J. A., Chapman, RC., Copplestone, A. A., Hamblin, T. J. & Oscier, D. G. (2000). VH gene status but not additional cytogenetic abnormalities predicts clinical outcome with CLL and trisomy 12. *Blood* **96**(Suppl.), 715a.

Houlston, R. S., Catovsky, D. & Yuille, M. R. (2002). Genetic susceptibility to chronic lymphocytic leukaemia. *Leukemia* **16**, 1008–1014.

Huang, Y. Q. Raphael, B., Buchbinder, A., Li, J. J., Zhang, W. G. & Friedman-Kien, A. E. (1994). Rearrangement and expression of MDM_2 oncogene in chronic lymphocytic leukemia. *American Journal of Hematology* **47**, 139–141.

Hultdin, M., Rjosenquist, R., Thunberg, U., Tobin, G., Norrback, K. F., Johnson, A., Sundstrom, C. & Roos, G. (2003). Association between telomere length and V_H gene mutation status in chronic lymphocytic leukaemia: clinical and biological implications. *British Journal of Cancer* **88**, 593–598.

Hurley, J. N., Man Fu, S., Kunkel, H. G., Chaganti, R. S. K. & German, J. (1980). Chromosome abnormalities of leukaemic B lymphocytes in chronic lymphocytic leukaemia. *Nature* **283**, 76–78.

Juliusson, G., Friberg, K. & Gahrton, G. (1988). Consistency of chromosomal aberrations in chronic B-lymphocytic leukemia. *Cancer* **62**, 500–506.

Juliusson, G., Oscier, D. G., Fitchett, M., Ross, F. M., Stockdill, G., Mackie, M. J., Parker, A. C., Castoldi G. L., Cuneo A., Knuutila S. and 2 others (1990). Prognostic subgroups in B-cell chronic lymphocytic leukemia defined by specific chromosomal abnormalities. *New England Journal of Medicine* **323**, 720–724.

Juliusson, G., Gahrton, G., Oscier, D., Fitchett, M., Ross, F., Brito-Babapulle, V., Catovsky, D., Knuutila, S., Elonen, E., Lechleitner, M. and 7 others (1991). Cytogenetic findings and survival in B-cell chronic lymphocytic leukemia. Second IWCCLL compilation of data on 662 patients. *Leukemia and Lymphoma* (Suppl.), 21–25.

Kalachikov, S., Migliazza, A., Cayanis, E., Fracchiolla, N. S., Bonaldo, M. F., Lawton, L., Jelenc, P., Ye, X., Qu, X., Chien, M. and 14 others (1997). Cloning and gene mapping of the chromosome 13q14 region deleted in chronic lymphocytic leukemia. *Genomics* **42**, 369–377.

Kapanadze, B., Kashuba, V., Baranova, A., Rasool, O., van Everdink, W., Liu, Y., Syomov, A., Corcoran, M., Poltaraus, A. Brodyansky, V. and 17 others (1998). A cosmid and cDNA fine physical map of a human chromosome 13q14 region frequently lost in B-cell chronic lymphocytic leukemia and identification of a new putative tumour suppressor gene, Leu 5. *FEBS Letters* **426**, 266–270.

Kapanadze, B., Makeevaa, N., Corcoran, M. M., Jareborg, N., Hammarsund, M., Baranova, A. Zabarovsky, E., Vorontcova, O., Merup, M., Jansson, O. and 5 others (2000). Comparative sequence analysis of a region on human chromosome 13q14, frequently deleted in B-cell chronic lymphocytic leukemia and its homologous region on mouse chromosome 14. *Blood* **96**(Suppl. 1), 703a.

Knuutila, S., Elonen, E., Teerenhovi, L., Rossi, L., Leskinen, R., Bloomfield, CD. & de la Chapelle, A. (1986). Trisomy 12 in B cells of patients with B-cell chronic lymphocytic leukemia. *New England Journal of Medicine* **314**, 865–869.

Krober, A., Seiler, T., Leupolt, E., Dohner, H. & Stilgenbauer S. (2000). IgVH mutated and unmutated B-CLL tumors show distinct genetic aberration patterns. *Blood* **96**(Suppl. 1) 835a.

Krober, A., Seiler, T., Benner, A., Bullinger, L., Breuckle, E., Lichter, P., Dohner, H. & Stilgenbauer, S. (2002). V_H mutation status, CD38 expression level, genomic aberrations and survival in chronic lymphocytic leukaemia. *Blood* **100**, 1410–1416.

Larramendy, M. L., Slitonen, S. M., Zhu, A., Hurme, M., Vilpo, L., Vilpo, J. A. & Knuutila, S. (1998). Optimized mitogen stimulation indices proliferation of neoplastic B cells in chronic lymphocytic leukemia: significance for cytogenetic analysis. *Cytogenetics and Cell Genetics* **82**, 215–221.

Lee, J., Giles, F., Huh, Y., Manshouri, T., O'Brien, S., Kantarjian, M., Keating, M. & Albitar, M. (2003). Molecular differences between small and large cells in patients with chronic lymphocytic leukaemia. *European Journal of Haematology* **71**, 235–242.

Lens, D., Dyer, M. J. S., Garcia-Marco, J. M., De Schouwer, P. J. J. C., Hamoudi, R. A., Jones, D., Farahat, N., Matutes, E. & Catovsky, D. (1997). p53 abnormalities in CLL are associated with excess of prolymphocytes and poor prognosis. *British Journal of Haematology* **99**, 848–857.

Lichter, P., Joos, S., Bentz, M. & Lampel, S. (2000). Comparative genomic hybridization: uses and limitations. *Seminars in Haematology* **37**, 348–357.

Lin, K., Sherrington, P. D., Dennis, M., Matrai, Z., Cawley, J. C. & Pettitt, A. R. (2002). Relationship between p53 dysfunction, CD38 expression, and IgV(H) mutation in chronic lymphocytic leukaemia. *Blood* **100**, 1404–1409.

Liu Y., Corcoran, M., Rasool, O., Ivanova, G., Ibbotson, R., Grander, D., Iyengar, A., Baranova, A., Kashuba, V., Merup, M. and 14 others (1997). Cloning of two candidate tumor suppressor genes within a 10 kb region on chromosome 13q14 frequently deleted in chronic lymphocytic leukemia. *Oncogene* **15**, 2463–2473.

Martens, U. M., Brass, V., Sedlacek, L., Pantic, M., Exner, C., Guo, Y., Engelhardt, M., Lansdorp, P.M., Waller, C. F. & Lange, W. (2002). Telomere maintenance in human B lymphocytes. *British Journal of Haematology* **119**, 810–818.

Matolcsy A., Inghirami G. & Knowles D. M. (1994). Molecular genetic demonstration of the diverse evolution of Richter's syndrome (chronic lymphocytic leukemia and subsequent large cell lymphoma). *Blood* **83**, 1363–1372.

McKeithan, T. W., Takimoto, G. S., Ohno, H., Bjorling, V. S., Morgan, R., Hecht, B. K., Dube, I., Sandberg, A. A. & Rowley, J. D. (1997). *BCL3I* rearrangements and t(14;19) in chronic lymphocytic leukemia and other B-cell malignancies: a molecular and cytogenetic study. *Genes, Chromosomes and Cancer* **20**, 64–72.

Mertens, D., Wolf, S., Schroeter, P., Schaffner, C., Dohner, H., Stilgenbauer, S. & Lichter, P. (2002). Down-regulation of candidate tumor suppressor genes within chromosome band 13q14.3 is independent of the DNA methylation pattern in B-cell chronic lymphocytic leukaemia. *Blood* **99**, 4116–4121.

Merup, M., Moreno, T. C., Heyman, M., Ronnberg, K., Grander, D., Detlofsson, R., Rasool, O., Liu, Y., Soderhall, S., Juliusson, G. and 2 others (1998a). 6q deletions in acute lymphoblastic leukemia and non-Hodgkin's lymphomas. *Blood* **91**, 3397–3400.

Merup, M., Jansson, M., Corcoran, M., Liu, Y., Wu, X., Rasool, O., Stellan, B., Hermansson, M., Juliussson, G., Gahrton, G. & Einhorn, S. (1998b). A FISH cosmid 'cocktail' for detection of 13q deletions in chronic lymphocytic leukaemia – comparison with cytogenetics and Southern hybridization. *Leukemia* **12**, 705–709.

Michaux, L., Dierlamm, J., Wlodarska, I., Bours, V., Van den Berghe, H. & Hagemeijer, A. (1997). t(14;19)/BCL3 rearrangements in lymphoproliferative disorders: A review of 23 cases. *Cancer Genetics and Cytogenetics* **94**, 36–43.

Migliazza, A., Bosch, F., Komatsu, H., Cayanis, E., Martinotti, S., Toniato, E., Guccione, E., Qu, X., Chien, M., Murty, V. V. V. and 9 others (2001). Nucleotide sequence, transcription map, and mutation analysis of the 13q14 chromosomal region deleted in B-cell chronic lymphocytic leukemia. *Blood* **97**, 2098–2104.

Neilson, J. R., Auer, R., White, D., Bienz, N., Waters, J. J., Whittaker, J. A., Milligan, D. W. & Fegan, C. D. (1997). Deletions at 11q identify a subset of patients with typical CLL who show consistent disease progression and reduced survival. *Leukemia* **11**, 1929–1932.

O'Connor, S. J. M., Su'ut, L., Morgan, G. J. & Jack, A. S. (2000). The relationship between typical and atypical B-cell chronic lymphocytic leukemia. A comparative genomic hybridization based study. *American Journal of Clinical Pathology* **114**, 448–458.

Ohno, H., Doi, S., Yabumoto, K., Fukuhara, S. & McKeithan, T. W. (1993). Molecular characterization of the t(14;19)(q32;q13)translocation in chronic lymphocytic leukemia. *Leukemia* **7**, 2057–2063.

Oscier, D. (1994). Cytogenetic and molecular abnormalities in chronic lymphocytic leukaemia. *Blood Reviews* **8**, 88–97.

Oscier, D. G., Matutes, E., Copplestone, A., Pickering, R. M., Chapman, R., Gillingham, R., Catovsky, D. & Hamblin, T. J. (1997). Atypical lymphocyte morphology: an adverse prognostic factor for disease progression in stage A CLL independent of trisomy 12. *British Journal of Haematology* **98**, 934–939.

Oscier, D. G., Gardiner, A. C., Mould, S. J., Glide, S., Davis, Z., Ibbottson, R. E., Corcoran, M. M., Chapman, R. M., Thomas, P. W., Copplestone, J. A. and 2 others (2002). Multivariate analysis of prognostic factors in CLL: clinical stage, IGVH gene mutational status, and loss or mutation of the p53 gene are independent prognostic factors. *Blood* **100**, 1177–1184.

Perez-Losada, A., Wessman, M., Tiainen, M., Hopman, A. H. N., Williard, H. F., Sole, F., Caballin, M. R., Woessner, S. & Knuutila, S. (1991). Trisomy 12 in chronic lymphocytic leukemia: an interphase cytogenetic study. *Blood* **78**, 775–779.

Pettitt, A. R., Sherrington, P. D., Cawley, J. C. (1999). The effect of p53 dysfunction on purine analogue cytotoxicity in chronic lymphocytic leukaemia. *British Journal of Haematology* **106**, 1049–1051.

Pettitt, A. R., Sherrington, P. D., Stewart, G., Cawley, J. C., Taylor, M. R. & Stankovic, T. (2001). p53 dysfunction in B-cell chronic lymphocytic leukaemia: inactivation of ATM as an alternative to TP53 mutation. *Blood* **98**, 814–822.

Que, T. H., Garcia-Marco, J., Ellis, J., Matutes, E., Brito Babapulle, V., Boyle, S. & Catovsky, D. (1993). Trisomy 12 in chronic lymphocytic leukemia detected by fluorescence in situ hybridization: analysis by stage, immunophenotype and morphology. *Blood* **82**, 571–575.

Qian, L., Gong, J., Liu, J., Broome, J. D. & Koduru, P. R. K. (1999). Cyclin D2 promoter disrupted by t(12;22)(p13;q11.2) during transformation of chronic lymphocytic leukaemia to non Hodgkin's lymphoma. *British Journal of Haematology* **106**, 477–485.

Santulli, B., Kazmierczak, B., Napolitano, R., Caliendo, I., Chiappetta, G., Rippe, V., Bullerdiek, J. & Fusco, A. (2000). A 12q13 translocation involving the *HMG1-C* gene in Richter transformation of a chronic lymphocytic leukemia. *Cancer Genetics and Cytogenetics* **119**, 70–73.

Satterwhite, E. D., Sonoki, T., Willis, T. G., Harder, L., Nowak, R., Arriola, E. L., Liu, H., Price, H. P., Gesk, S., Steinemann, D., Schlegelberger, B., Oscier, D. G., Siebert, R., Tucker, P. W. & Dyer, M. J. S. (2001). The BCL11 gene family: involvement of BCL11A in lymphoid malignancies. *Blood* **98**, 3413–3420.

Schaffner, C., Stilgenbauer, S., Rappold, G. A., Dohner, H. & Lichter, P. (1999). Somatic *ATM* mutations indicate a pathogenic role of ATM in B-cell chronic lymphocytic leukemia. *Blood* **94**, 748–753.

Schaffner, C., Scheuermann, M., Kalla, J., Dohner, H., Stilgenbauer, S. & Lichter, P. (2000). Analysis of *PPP2R1B.*, a candidate tumor suppressor gene at 11q22-q23, in B-CLL. *Blood* **96**(Suppl. 2), 175b.

Schmidt, H. H., Dyomin, V., Palanisamy, N., Nanjangud, G., Pirc-Danoewinata, H., Haas, O. A. & Chaganti, R. S. K. (2000). Dysregulation of the chrondroitin 4–0 sulfotransferase 1, (*C4ST-1*) gene by a t(12;14)(q23;q32) in a case of B-cell chronic lymphocytic leukemia (B-CLL). *Blood* **96**(Suppl. 2), 161b.

Stankovic, T., Weber, P., Stewart, G., Bedenham, T., Murray, J., Byrd, P. J., Moss, P. A. H. & Taylor, A. M. R. (1999). Inactivation of ataxia telangiectasia mutated gene in B-cell chronic lymphocytic leukaemia. *The Lancet* **353**, 26–29.

Stankovic, T., Stewart, G. S., Fegan, C., Biggs, P., Last, J., Byrd, P. J., Keenan, R. D., Moss, P. A. H. & Taylor, A. M. R. (2002). Ataxia telangiectasia mutated-deficient B-cell chronic lymphocytic leukaemia occurs in pregerminal center cells and results in defective damage response and unrepaired chromosome damage. *Blood* **99**, 300–309.

Stankovic, T., Hubank, M., Cronin, D., Stewart, G.S., Fletcher, D., Bignell, C.R., Alvi, A.J., Austen, B., Weston, V. J., Fegan, C., Byrd, P. J., Moss, P. A. H. & Taylor, A. M. R. (2004). Microarray analysis reveals that TP53 and ATM mutant B-CLLs share a defect in activation of pro-apoptotic responses following DNA damage but are distinguished by major differences in activation of pro-survival responses. *Blood* **103**, 291–300.

Starostick, P., Manshouri, T., O'Brien, S., Freireich, E., Kantarjian, H., Haidar, M., Lerner, S., Keating, M. & Albitar, M. (1998). Deficiency of the ATM protein expression defines an aggressive subgroup of B-cell chronic lymphocytic leukemia. *Cancer Research* **20**, 2552–4557.

Stilgenbauer, S., Liebisch, P., James, M. R., Schroder, M., Schlegelberger, B., Fischer, K., Bentz, M., Lichter, P. & Dohner, H. (1996). Molecular cytogenetic delineation of a novel critical genomic region in chromosome bands 11q22.3–923.1 in lymphoproliferative disorders. *Proceedings of the National Academy of Sciences of the United States of America* **93**, 11,837–11,841.

Stilgenbauer, S., Nickolenko, J., Wilhelm, J., Wolf, S., Weitz, S., Dohner, K., Boehm, T., Dohner, H. & Lichter P. (1998). Expressed sequences as candidates for a novel tumor suppressor gene at band 13q14 in B-cell chronic lymphocytic leukemia and mantle cell lymphoma. *Oncogene* **14**, 1891–1897.

Stilgenbauer, S., Bullinger, L., Benner, A., Wildenberger, K., Bentz, M., Dohner, K., Ho, A. D., Lichter, P. & Dohner, H. (1999). Incidence and clinical significance of 6q deletions in B cell chronic lymphocytic leukemia. *Leukemia* **13**, 1331–1334.

Stilgenbauer, S., von Neuhoff, N., Bullinger, L., Krober, A., Lichter, P., Dreger, P. & Dohner, H. (2000). Deletion 11q23 indentifies B-CLL patients at high risk for molecular disease persistence after high dose therapy and autografting. *Blood* **96**(Suppl. 1), 715a.

Stilgenbauer, S. (2003a). V_H mutation status and genomic aberrations in the clinical risk assessment of CLL. *Leukemia and Lymphoma* **44** (Suppl. 2), S7–S8.

Stilgenbauer, S., Winkler, D., Kienle, D., Krober, A., Emmerick, B., Hallek, M. & Doehner, H. (2003b). CLL2H protocol of the German CLL Study Group (GCLLSG): subcutaneous Campath-1H (MabCampath) in fludarabine-refractory CLL. *Leukemia and Lymphoma* **44** (Suppl. 2), S48.

Stratowa, C., Loffler, G., Lichter, P., Stilgenbauer, S., Haberl, P., Schweifer, N. Dohner, H. & Wilgenbus, K. K.(2001). cDNA microarray gene expression analysis of B-cell chronic lymphocytic leukemia proposes potential new prognostic markers involved in lymphocytic trafficking. *International Journal of Cancer* **91**, 474–480.

Thornton, P. D., Matutes, E., Bosanquet, A. G., Lakhani, A. K., Grech, H., Ropner, J. E., Joshi, R., Mackie, P. H., Douglas, I. D., Bowcock, S. J. & Catovsky, D. (2003). High dose methylprednisolone can induce remissions in CLL patients with p53 abnormalities. *Annals of Hematology* **82**, 759–765.

Van Everdink, W., Baranova, A., Lummen, C., Tyazhelova, T., Looman, M., Ivanov, D., Verlind, E., Pestova, A., Faber, H., van der Veen, A. and 3 others (2003). RFP2, c13ORF1, and FAM10A4 are the most likely tumour suppressor gene candidates for B-cell chronic lymphocytic leukaemia. *Cancer Genetics and Cytogenetics* **146**, 48–57.

Voss, T., Ahorn, H., Haberl, P., Dohner, H. & Wilgenbus, K.(2001). Correlation of clinical data with proteomics profiles in 24 patients with B-cell chronic lymphocytic leukemia. *International Journal of Cancer* **91**, 180–186.

Watanabe, T., Hotta, T., Ichikawa, A., Kinoshita, T., Nagai, H., Uchida, T., Murate, T. & Saito, H. (1994). The *MDM2* oncogene overexpression in chronic lymphocytic leukemia and low-grade lymphoma of B-cell origin. *Blood* **84**, 3158–3165.

Wattel, E., Preudhomme, C., Hecquet, B., Vanrumbeke, M., Quesnel, B., Dervite, I., Morel, P. & Fenaux, P. (1994). p53 mutations are associated with resistance to chemotherapy and short survival in hematologic malignancies. *Blood* **84**, 3148–3157.

Zhu, Y., Monni, O., El-Rifai, W., Siitonen, SM., Vilpo, L., Vilpo, J. & Knuutila, S. (1999). Discontinuous deletions at 11q23 in B cell chronic lymphocytic leukemia. *Leukemia* **13**, 708–712.

Chapter 3

Natural history of chronic lymphocytic leukaemia: current thinking

Andrew R. Pettitt, Paul D. Sherrington, David J. Allsup, Zoltan Matrai, John C. Cawley and Mirko Zuzel

Introduction

It has long been recognised that chronic lymphocytic leukaemia (CLL) is a very heterogeneous disease in terms of its clinical presentation and kinetics. Here we review recent findings that offer some insights into the origin of the disease and the biological basis of this heterogeneity. The issues that will be addressed are outlined in Table 3.1.

Table 3.1 Topics of current interest relevant for the evolution and progression of CLL

- V_H mutation
- p53/ATM
- CD38
- Routes of development and role of antigen
- BCR function
- Microenvironmental interactions
- Tissue homing
- Deregulated immunity

V_H mutation and its relevance to CLL

It is now uncontroversial that the degree of mutation of the immunoglobulin (Ig) heavy chain V gene (V_H) varies considerably in CLL (Fais *et al.* 1998), and that patients with extensively mutated V_H genes have a better prognosis than those with less V_H mutation (Damle *et al.* 1999; Hamblin *et al.* 1999). This led to the concept that CLL might be two diseases: one derived from 'mutated' (M) post-germinal centre memory B cells, the other from 'unmutated' (UM) pre-germinal centre B cells (Naylor & Capra 1999). Although this theory has been largely ruled out by the discovery that the gene expression profiles of both M and UM CLL cells are very similar to that of normal memory B cells (Klein *et al.* 2001; Rosenwald *et al.* 2001), the idea persists that CLL is separable into two biologically distinct prognostic groups defined by V_H mutational status (Kay *et al.* 2002).

Definition of M- and UM-subgroups

When separating CLL patients according to V_H mutation, a cut-off value of 2% has historically been used on the theoretical grounds that minor divergences from the nearest published germline sequence might, in some patients, be due to the expression of previously unrecognised unmutated polymorphic V_H variants (Damle *et al.* 1999; Hamblin *et al.* 1999). This approach is, of course, a compromise because some polymorphisms may differ from the germline sequence by >2%, whereas some somatic mutations are likely to result in <2% divergence. Clearly, as the databases become ever more comprehensive, the chance of mistaking polymorphisms for mutations becomes increasingly unlikely and the need for a threshold on theoretical grounds correspondingly less valid. More recently, attempts have been made to define the most appropriate V_H mutation cut-off on the more pragmatic basis of patient survival. Statistical methods that identify the best compromise between sensitivity and specificity in recognising poor prognosis patients have been applied to two large series of patients and have yielded optimal cut-off values of between 2% and 4% (Kröber *et al.* 2001, 2002; Oscier *et al.* 2002).

Compared with other biological prognostic factors, V_H mutational status seems to be a particularly good determinant of long, but not short, survival. For example, in the original study of Hamblin *et al.* (1999), the median disease-specific survival of patients with M- and UM-CLL defined by a 2% cut-off was about 25 and 8 years, respectively. Interestingly, in a subsequent report (Oscier *et al.* 2002), the same group found that a threshold value of 5% defined a poor-risk UM group with maximal sensitivity (and therefore a corresponding good-risk M group with maximum specificity). In keeping with this, we found that the survival of patients with 2-5% V_H mutation was significantly shorter than that of patients with >5% mutation (Lin *et al.* 2002). We also showed that two other adverse prognostic factors – p53 dysfunction and CD38 expression – occurred almost exclusively among patients with <5% V_H mutation (Figure 3.1). Other reports have detected less precise associations between UM-CLL and CD38 expression, p53 abnormalities and adverse karyotype, but these studies have classified cases into M versus UM on the basis of lower threshold values of V_H mutation (Oscier *et al.* 2002; Kröber *et al.* 2002). It seems, therefore, that most CLL patients with >5% mutation have an extremely benign form of the disease, whereas patients with <5% mutation display considerable heterogeneity (Figure 3.2).

Possible explanations for the poor outcome of UM-CLL

The poor prognosis of patients with UM V_H genes may be partly explained by an increased frequency of p53 dysfunction, adverse cytogenetics and CD38 expression. However, UM-CLL is also associated with other factors that may affect the biology of the malignant cells. For example, activation-induced cytidine deaminase (AID) is more readily detectable in UM- than M-CLL clones (McCarthy *et al.* 2003; Albesiano *et al.* 2003). AID is involved in DNA recombination and SHM and may therefore

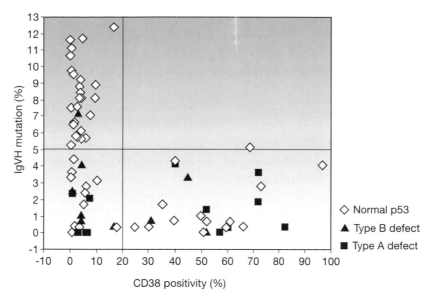

Figure 3.1 Relationship between extent of IgV$_H$ mutation, CD38 positivity and p53 dysfunction. Results are shown from 83 CLL patients attending the Royal Liverpool University Hospital. Note that almost every patient with >20% CD38 positivity or p53 dysfunction had <5% V$_H$ mutation. Patients with p53 dysfunction are indicated by closed symbols. Type A p53 dysfunction is associated with p53 mutation, whereas the type B defect results from ATM mutation (see Figure 3.3).

provide a background of genomic instability that facilitates the evolution of CLL clones with mutations conferring a proliferation and/or survival advantage. In addition, UM-CLL clones tend to generate stronger signals after B-cell receptor (BCR) ligation (Lanham *et al.* 2003; Allsup *et al.* 2002). *In vivo*, such BCR responsiveness may result in tumour-cell proliferation and protection from apoptosis. Interestingly, gene expression profiling showed that UM-CLL is associated with increased levels of mRNA encoding the ZAP-70 tyrosine kinase (Klein *et al.* 2001; Rosenwald *et al.* 2001), which may potentiate signalling through the BCR (Chen *et al.* 2002). Subsequent work has shown that ZAP-70 mRNA levels correlate well with protein expression, and that the latter has prognostic value (Wiestner *et al.* 2003). Recently, FACS methods for measuring ZAP-70 have been developed that appear to be as effective as V$_H$ mutation in separating patients into good (ZAP-70+) and bad (ZAP-70–) prognostic groups (Crespo *et al.* 2003; Orchard *et al.* 2003).

The V$_H$-3-21 engima

The V$_H$3-21 gene segment is rarely expressed by normal B cells but frequently utilised in CLL, where it is associated with a distinctive CDR3 and preferential usage of V$_\lambda$2-14 (Tobin *et al.* 2002, 2003). Interestingly, V$_H$3-21 is also the most frequently

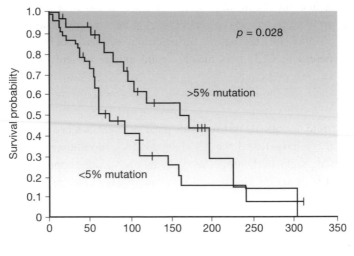

(a)

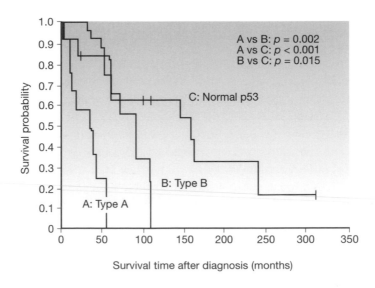

(b)

Figure 3.2 Prognostic effect of V_H mutation and p53 dysfunction. (a) Survival of patients according to V_H mutation using a 5% threshold value. (b) Survival of patients with <5% V_H mutation according to p53 status (see Figure 3.3).

utilised gene segment in the B cells of patients with rheumatoid arthritis, and V_H3-21-utilising B cells from such patients are capable of producing rheumatoid factor in vitro (He *et al.* 1995). In rheumatoid arthritis, V_H3-21 is usually in germline configuration, whereas in CLL it is mostly found among patients with >2% V_H mutation. However, despite being mostly 'mutated', CLL patients utilising V_H3-21 have a poor prognosis. (Tobin *et al.* 2002, 2003). No association has been observed in CLL between V_H3-21 usage and adverse karyotype (Kröber *et al.* 2002b), and the poor clinical outcome of patients utilising this gene segment has been considered an enigma. However, we have found that the extent of V_H mutation in our series of patients using this V_H segment did not exceed 5% and that a high proportion displayed p53 dysfunction (Lin *et al.* 2003). These two findings may therefore help to explain the bad prognosis of this subgroup of CLL.

p53/ATM inactivation

p53 gene abnormalities occur in about 10–15% of patients with CLL, the usual defect being mutation of one allele and deletion of the other at 17p13. These patients have a particularly aggressive form of the disease, characterised by chemo-resistance, prolymphocytic transformation, and a median survival of only 2–3 years (El Rouby *et al.* 1993; Wattel *et al.* 1994; Dohner *et al.* 1995, 2000; Lens *et al.* 1997; Cordone *et al* 1998; Oscier *et al.* 2002; Lin *et al.* 2002). This reflects the role of p53 in maintaining genomic integrity in the face of DNA damage by triggering apoptosis or by inducing cell-cycle arrest and DNA repair. Consequently, tumour cells with defective p53 undergo rapid clonal expansion, are resistant to chemotherapy and are highly prone to clonal evolution (Lane 1992; Vogelstein *et al.* 2000; Balint & Vousden 2001). In addition to detecting p53 mutations in about 15% of cases of CLL, we have also shown that a similar proportion have p53 dysfunction due to inactivation of ATM (Pettitt *et al.* 2001), a kinase encoded at 11q23 that phosphorylates p53 in response to double-strand DNA breaks (Stankovic *et al.* 2002a). Such patients also have an aggressive form of the disease with a median survival of about 6 years (Starostik *et al.* 1998; Bullrich *et al.* 1999; Stankovic *et al.* 1999; Lin *et al.* 2002). The precise relationship between ATM mutations and deletions of 11q23 is, as yet, unclear. It is also unclear at what point p53/ATM mutations/deletions are acquired during the development of CLL, although one report suggests that ATM mutation may occur prior to malignant transformation (Stankovic *et al.* 2002b). CLL clones with p53 or ATM mutations can be readily detected by virtue of their impaired p53 response to ionising radiation (Figure 3.3).

CD38

It is now firmly established that CD38 is an adverse prognostic indicator in CLL (Damle *et al.* 1999; Ibrahim *et al.* 2001), but exactly why this is so is still not clear. It is also now established that there is an imperfect relationship between CD38 and V_H

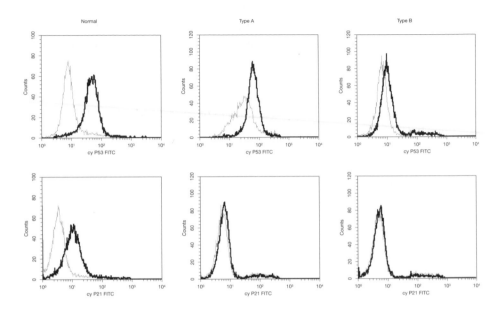

Figure 3.3 Clinical test for p53 dysfunction. Isolated CLL cells exposed to ionising radiation (IR), cultured overnight and analysed for the expression of p53 and one of its transcriptional targets, p21. FACS histograms show p53 and p21 expression in irradiated (red line) and non-irradiated (green line) cells. The normal response is characterised by IR-induced accumulation of both p53 and p21. In the type A defect associated with p53 mutation, basal levels of p53 are increased (mutant p53 has a prolonged half-life), and IR-induced p21 up-regulation is impaired. In the type B defect associated with ATM mutation, basal levels of p53 are not increased, but IR-induced accumulation of both p53 and p21 is impaired.

mutation in that most CD38$^+$ CLL clones have been found in the UM group. However, around half of the clones within this group are CD38$^-$ (Matrai *et al.* 2001).

CD38 positivity in the disease is usually assessed by measuring the number of CD19$^+$ B cells coexpressing CD38 at their cell surface. The detection of surface CD38 is critically dependent on the monoclonal antibody (Mab) used, and most studies have employed a Mab known as HB-7 (Damle *et al.* 1999; Hamblin *et al.* 1999). It is not known why different antibodies give different results for surface CD38 (sCD38). However, work from this laboratory indicates that CLL cells, like a range of other cell types, contain different multimeric forms of CD38 which are differentially recognised by the available antibodies. It is also not clear how many CLL cells should express sCD38 in a given case to regard it as 'CD38 positive' (Kröber *et al.* 2002a; Ghia *et al.* 2003). However, most studies have used a 'cut-off' of 20–30% CD19$^+$ CD38$^+$ cells (Damle *et al.* 1999; Ibrahim *et al* 2001; Lin *et al.* 2002).

During B-cell ontogeny, the expression of CD38 is tightly regulated. The protein is highly expressed by B-cell precursors and then becomes progressively reduced and finally absent on mature naïve cells. CD38 is then re-expressed during the cells' passage through germinal-centre maturation stages. Fully mature quiescent memory cells again lack protein expression but, on memory recall and maturation to plasma cells, CD38 again becomes strongly expressed (Konoplera *et al.* 2000). It is not clear what this tells us about the stage of differentiation of CD38$^+$ CLL clones. However, because CLL cells resemble memory cells in gene array studies, it may be that CD38$^+$ CLL clones represent antigen-activated memory cells that are beginning to differentiate towards plasma cells, but are blocked at a pre-plasma cell stage.

CD38 is a 45 kDa type II transmembrane ectoenzyme (Figure 3.4) that in different cell types tends to associate into covalently or non-covalently bound multimers. The ADP ribosyl cyclase activity of the molecule increases with the degree of multimerisation. It is, however, not known what molecular forms of CD38 are present in CLL cells, and the enzymatic activities of the molecule have not been studied in this cell type. However, it seems reasonable to presume that, by generating cyclic ADP ribose, CD38 participates in the regulation of a range of cellular functions controlled by cytosolic Ca^{2+} rises. For instance, it is known that CD38 influences CLL-cell signalling through the BCR (Zupo *et al.* 1996) and that the molecule is involved in the proliferation and survival of CLL cells (Deaglio *et al.* 2003). This latter involvement is likely to contribute to the increased tumour bulk that is a feature of progressive disease with an adverse prognosis.

In addition to having enzymatic activity, CD38 can also perform an adhesive receptor function by binding to PECAM (CD31) (Deaglio *et al.* 2000), an adhesion ligand present on several cell types including endothelial cells. The functional significance of this CD38-CD31 interaction for CLL cells is still unclear. However, because CD31 is important in transendothelial migration (TEM) (Worthylake & Burridge, 2001) and because CD38 is important for the motility of other cell types (Partida-Sanchez *et al.* 2001), it is tempting to speculate that CD38-CD31 interaction may play a role in the CLL-cell TEM important for malignant-cell invasion of lymphoreticular tissues. In this context, it has been reported that high CD38 expression is associated with lymphadenopathy (Ibrahim *et al.* 2001).

Routes of development of CLL clones and the role of antigen

Because CLL cells are CD5$^+$ it has long been assumed that they are related to the B1 subpopulation of normal B cells. These cells are now known to be positively selected by interaction with particular types of self-antigen during foetal and neonatal development. Although in adults B1 cells are predominantly peritoneal B cells, a similar type of cell is also found among marginal zone B cells (Dammers *et al.* 2000).

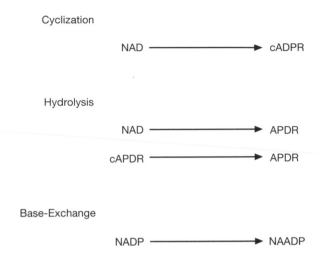

Figure 3.4 Reactions catalysed by CD38. cADPR & NAADP = cyclic ADP-ribose and nicotinic acid adenine dinucleotide phosphate respectively. Both cause Ca^{2+} release from intracellular stores.

Such marginal zone B cells provide a rapid immune response by secretion of IgM antibodies. These positively selected B cells have a particular affinity for T-dependent self/bacterial antigens and are currently regarded as part of the innate immune system (Bendelac *et al.* 2001; Marchalonis *et al.* 2002). It was initially thought that M-CLL clones are more mature cells responding to T-dependent antigens, whereas UM-CLL clones represent cells at a pre-germinal-centre stage of development. However, it is currently accepted that all CLL cell clones are memory-type cells (Klein *et al.* 2001) which are more or less activated. Thus, it appears that the cells giving rise to different CLL-cell clones have reached a similar maturation stage, but possibly by different routes of antigen-directed diversification. If this is the case, then the type of antigen and the extent of antigenic stimulation become principal factors which impact on disease heterogeneity and progression. Indeed, it is currently assumed that antigenic stimulation plays a central role in the selection and maturation of CLL cells (Fais *et al.* 1998; Damle *et al.* 2002), not only before, but possibly also after, their transformation into arrested, progressively accumulating cells.

Antigen in the selection and diversification of B cells to potential CLL-cell precursors

During normal B-cell development, the cells capable of providing effective immunity without harmful anti-self reactivity are generated in the process of antigen-driven selection and maturation. The potentially harmful cells are killed, i.e. negatively selected, at an immature stage by a high concentration of self-antigens. The surviving cells then further mature and diversify into cells that provide either innate immunity

(B1 cells and marginal zone (MZ) cells) or adaptive immunity (B2 cells, follicular (FO) B cells) (Xiaoli *et al.* 2001).

Cells providing innate immunity give rise to circulating IgD$^+$, CD27$^+$ memory cells that are the major source of secreted IgM (Shi *et al.* 2003). However, it should be noted that cells with such a phenotype can also be generated from naïve IgD$^-$, CD27$^-$ B2 cells at the germinal-centre founder stage of their response to T-dependent antigens (Bohnhorst *et al.* 2001). However, the principal long-lived memory cells generated during the latter response are IgD$^-$ CD27$^+$ cells that have undergone the germinal-centre reaction and express hypermutated, class-switched and affinity-selected immunoglobulin (Klein *et al.* 1997). Thus, assuming that somatic V_H gene mutation and class switch require a T-dependent germinal-centre response, V_H-gene UM CLL clones could potentially originate from innate immunity cells responding to T-independent antigens, or from germinal-centre founder cells that have undergone an incomplete T-dependent response. Mutated cells, on the other hand, could only correspond to cells that have responded to T-dependent antigens by a germinal-centre reaction, but have selectively failed to undergo class-switch recombination.

However, recent studies clearly show that the above assumption linking Ig hyper-mutation and class-switch exclusively to T-dependent germinal-centre B-cell development is incorrect. Thus, V_H-gene mutation can occur in the absence of T-cell help and germinal-centre formation (de Vinuesa *et al.* 2000; Weller *et al.* 2001; Euler *et al.* 2002) opening the possibility that M-CLL clones may also originate from innate immunity cells that recognise T-independent antigens. Clearly, more knowledge regarding the correspondence between CLL-cell phenotype and the phenotypes of normal B cells responding to T-dependent versus T-independent antigens is required to resolve the question of the precise origin of CLL cells. Nevertheless, some insights into the nature of CLL cells and factors that may be important for disease progression may be obtained from CLL clones expressing BCRs with established specificities.

Type of antigen and its potential role in the selection and expansion of CLL-cell clones

One of the indicators of antigen-driven B-cell selection is the biased usage of Ig gene segments which, in both M- and UM-CLL cells, often results in the creation of a BCR with a broad specificity and relatively low affinity for T-independent antigens (Shokri *et al.* 1993; Pritsch *et al.* 1993; Chiorazzi & Ferrarini 2003; Nollet *et al.* 2002; Potter *et al.* 2003). Triggering of the initial humoral response to such antigens does not require T-cell help and is mediated by IgM-secreting cells upon activation of IgD$^+$ CD27$^+$ memory cells of MZ origin belonging to the innate immune system (Martin & Kearney 2000). Later, when these complex antigens are processed by phagocytic antigen-presenting cells and the peptides from their protein-components presented to T cells, the innate response is joined by an adaptive response of follicular B cells that undergo the geminal-centre reaction to produce high-affinity class-switched antibodies (Martin *et al.* 2001; Lucas *et al.* 2001). This normally results in the effective clearance of the antigen that then terminates the response.

An important property of innate-immunity B cells is that they are positively selected by low concentrations of self-antigens with a structure that corresponds to, or mimics, that of some microbial constituents. Therefore, a break of tolerance to such self-antigen results in autoimmune diseases dominated by the generation and tissue-deposition of immune complexes. In several such conditions (e.g. rheumatoid arthritis, Sjogren's syndome and mixed cryoglobulinaemia) B cells secrete rheumatoid factor (RF) which is an antibody directed against the Fc portion of Ig bound to the microbial or self-antigens of a particular repetitive structure. Thus the cells with RF specificity, including many CLL-cell clones will, upon interaction with such antibody-coated antigen, receive a potent type 2 T-independent stimulus through extensive cross-linking of their BCR (Newkirk 2002).

In contrast to normal B lymphocytes, CLL cells will fail to respond to such stimuli by differentiating into antibody-secreting cells because of their maturational arrest. Moreover, because of the decline in adaptive immunity with advanced age (Johnson *et al* 2002), and the absence of secreted IgM to bridge the innate to the adaptive response, the patient may also fail to mount an effective T-dependent response to clear the antigen and thus protect CLL cells from chronic antigenic stimulation. Since such stimulation may drive CLL-cell proliferation, an effective adaptive response might provide a crucial degree of protection from clonal expansion of terminally-differentiation-arrested CLL cells.

The above sequence of events is supported by the prevalence of CLL in males (Damle *et al.* 1999), who seem to be less capable than females of mounting such adaptive responses, as shown by the distinctly higher incidence of autoimmune diseases caused by high anti-self-antibody production in women as compared with men (Newkirk 2002). It has been suggested that this sex-linked difference in mounting humoral T-dependent autoimmune responses reflects differential influences of oestrogen and testosterone on immune-response polarisation towards TH-2 and TH-1 type cytokine production (Wilder 1998; Huber *et al.* 1999).

The proposed importance of chronic antigenic stimulation in the pathogenesis of CLL implies a malignant-cell-specific breakdown of immune tolerance in which increased antigenic load, resulting from failure of these cells to produce antibodies that could clear/neutralise the antigen, might be only one of several contributing factors. For instance, the apparent terminal-differentiation block could itself keep the cells at a stage where they are intrinsically less prone to die and/or are protected from apoptosis by environmental factors including antigen, accessory cells and cytokines. Moreover, there is a wealth of literature describing a large spectrum of abnormalities of CLL cells and other cells of the immune system that could contribute to the pathogenesis of CLL, and also explain the well-recognised general deregulation of the immune system in this disease.

BCR function

Because CLL cells do not spontaneously proliferate, their clonal expansion in vivo must be driven by stimuli that may or may not originate from their direct interaction with antigen. In vitro, BCR cross-linking on its own can either kill CLL cells (Zupo *et al.* 2000), or promote their survival (Bernal *et al.* 2001), without triggering either cell proliferation or antibody secretion. Moreover, direct measurements of generated signals have shown that BCR translocation into lipid rafts (Allsup *et al.* 2002), cytosolic Ca^{2+} rise, protein tyrosine phosphorylation and ERK activation (Zupo *et al.* 2000; Allsup *et al.* 2002; Lanham *et al.* 2003) readily occur upon cross-linking of the BCR on UM, but not, M-CLL-cell clones. In addition, such cross-linking prolonged the survival of UM clones without having an obvious effect on the survival of M cells (Allsup *et al.* 2002).

It can therefore be tentatively concluded that UM-CLL cells will more readily respond to *in vivo* antigenic stimulation, and that this may indeed promote clonal expansion of these cells by prolonging their survival and, in the presence of co-stimuli, perhaps promote their proliferation. In contrast, the cells of M clones could be either intrinsically more resistant to stimulation of the BCR, or have become resistant following such stimulation. Whatever proves to be the case, these differences in BCR signalling observed between malignant cells from two different prognostic groups of CLL underscore the potential key role of antigenic stimulation in the generation and expansion of CLL-cell clones.

Microenvironmental interactions

Because of the differentiation block of CLL-cells and their clear dependence on external stimuli for proliferation and survival, the possible contribution of environmental stimuli to the pathogenesis of CLL has inevitably attracted a great deal of attention.

CLL is characterised by several abnormalities in the responses of malignant B cells and of accessory dendritic- and T-cells to stimuli that are either triggered by direct cell-cell contacts or depend on the production and secretion of cytokines. However, because of the two-way nature of such responses, it is often difficult to assess which of the reported abnormalities contribute to the clonal expansion of CLL-cells, and which are the consequence of this expansion. Moreover, even when the impact of age and sex on the immune system is taken into account, a comparative assessment of the real extent of any such abnormality is hampered by the fact that the true normal counterpart of CLL-cells has not yet been clearly identified, and may be different in different CLL cases.

Because the role of cytokines and accessory cells in the pathogenesis of CLL has already been comprehensively reviewed (Orsini *et al.* 2000), the following is only a limited selection of the reports that exemplify the work that has been performed in this field.

T-cell help has been considered as being important for development of CLL by supporting malignant-cell survival through a direct cell-cell interaction via CD40-CD40L (Furman *et al.* 2000) and also through IL2, IL-4 or IFN-γ production. On the other hand, abnormalities in cytotoxic T-cell generation in CLL have been described that could be partly attributed to advanced patient's age (Fagnoni *et al.* 2000) and partly induced by CLL cells, through either direct cell-cell interaction (Cantwell *et al.* 1997; Cerutti *et al.* 2001) or through TGFβ and/or IL-10 production (Schuler *et al.* 1999; Fillatreau *et al.* 2002; Scrivener *et al.* 2003). These abnormalities, combined with an inefficient antigen presentation by both CLL cells (Dazzi *et al.* 1995) and dendritic cells (Orsini *et al.* 2003), are apparently important for the protection of CLL cells from the elimination by cytotoxic T cells. This protection, however, can be overcome by transfecting CLL cells with CD40L to induce homotypic CD40-CD40L interaction, and thus generate the stimulus for an increased presentation by the malignant cells of antigen(s) that can generate specific T-cell-dependent responses (Wierda *et al.* 2000).

Tissue homing

The pathogenetic importance of the tendency of CLL-cells to infiltrate bone marrow and secondary lymphoid tissues is uncontroversial. These tissues provide niches for malignant-cell proliferation and an environment that promotes cell survival.

In early stage CLL, the abnormal lymphocytes have a propensity to remain localised in the blood. Only in later stages of the disease do the malignant cells show a tendency to invade lymph nodes and accumulate therein. Also, heavy bone marrow involvement with impairment of normal haematopoiesis is a feature of advanced disease. Both processes are associated with a poor prognosis. Therefore, the mechanisms determining CLL-cell invasion of, and accumulation in, lymphoreticular tissues including bone marrow are of considerable clinical importance.

Normal lymphocyte homing is the result of cell migration into and within tissues – processes controlled by a range of adhesion receptors and chemokines. Selectivity and flexibility in normal lymphocyte homing is brought about by regulated expression of adhesion and chemokine receptors in different lymphocyte subsets and by the differential tissue distribution of adhesive ligands and chemokines (Sallusto *et al.* 2000). Normal lymphocyte extravasation involves adhesion to, and migration across, endothelium and its basement membrane. Initially, interaction between lymphocyte selectins and their carbohydrate ligands allows rolling on vascular endothelium. This allows the exposure of lymphocyte chemokine receptors to their ligands displayed on the surface of endothelial cells. Engagement of chemokine receptors induces rapid inside-out activation of integrins, firm adhesion and transmigration. Having extravasated, lymphocytes are then directed to specific sites within secondary lymphoid organs by processes controlled by chemokines and their receptors and by different extracellular matrix components within these organs.

We and others have defined some of the mechanisms involved in these processes in CLL.

Transendothelial migration (TEM) is essential for both entry into, and exit from, lymphoreticular tissues and is impaired in CLL (Chen *et al.* 1999). Regarding the specific mechanisms involved, CLL cells variably express L-selectin (CD62L) (Till *et al.* 2001) but there is no correlation between such expression and either TEM in vitro or clinical lymphadenopathy (Till *et al.* 2001). CLL cells variably express a range of other adhesion receptors. Important among these are $\alpha_4\beta_1$ and $\alpha_L\beta_2$ because both these integrin heterodimers are important for CLL-cell TEM (Till *et al.* 2001). Only in a proportion of CLL patients do the malignant cells possess $\alpha_4\beta_1$ and such expression is important for TEM and lymphadenopathy since CLL cells lacking $\alpha_4\beta_1$ are unable to undergo TEM in vitro and because blocking the interaction of α_4 with its ligand VCAM inhibits this process (Till *et al.* 2001). Furthermore, there is a strong correlation between $\alpha_4\beta_1$ expression and clinical lymphadenopathy (Till *et al.* 2001). It is not known why the abnormal cells from only a proportion of cases (~40%) express $\alpha_4\beta_1$. $\alpha_L\beta_2$ is also important in TEM in that blocking antibodies inhibits TEM *in vitro* (Till *et al.* 2001).

Regarding chemokines and their receptors, CLL cells possess a range of receptors and produce at least two chemokines (IL-8 and MIG) (di Celle *et al.* 1996; Jones *et al.* 2000). CLL cells can migrate in response to a number of chemokines, but the pathophysiological significance of such movement is often unclear. SDF-1 (CXCL12) and its receptor may be important for CLL-migration into and within bone marrow (Burger *et al.* 1999). We have shown that the expression of CCR7 varies from case to case and that CCR7 ligands (CCL19 and 21) can induce CLL-cell TEM; furthermore, there is some correlation in CLL between CCR7 expression and lymphadenopathy (Till *et al.* 2001). Therefore, it seems that expression of both $\alpha_4\beta_1$ and CCR7 influences the ability of CLL cells to undergo TEM and that the presence of both receptors correlates with clinical lymphadenopathy.

Once CLL cells have entered lymphoreticular tissues, their further migration and homing are presumably determined by gradients of different chemokines and by the adhesive ligands encountered in different areas. The precise processes involved are still largely unexplored, but we have shown that IL-8 and hyaluronan may be involved (Till *et al.* 1999). Hyaluronan is a glycosaminoglycan which is widely distributed in tissue extracellular matrix. Within lymphoreticular tissues, HA is abundant within the interfollicular areas of lymph nodes and in the white pulp of spleen, but is largely absent form the red pulp of this organ (Till *et al.* 1999). We have shown that CLL cells become motile on HA when stimulated with exogenous IL-8 and have demonstrated abundant IL-8 within CLL nodes (Till *et al.* 1999). It therefore seems likely that CLL-cell interaction with HA and IL-8 at least partly influences the homing of the cells within nodes. Also, the absence of HA from the red pulp of the spleen may be relevant to the fact that CLL cells do not infiltrate this area of the organ to any major extent. It is not known how other chemokines affect the movement of CLL cells on HA.

In addition to HA, a number of other adhesive ligands including collagen and fibronectin are present in lymphoreticular tissues. Despite often possessing the relevant integrin receptors for these ligands, CLL cells are usually poorly adherent to collagen- or fibronectin-coated surfaces and are not spontaneously motile on such surfaces (Vincent *et al.* 1996). This presumably indicates that the integrins of CLL cells are usually not activated and require stimulation for inside-out activation. It remains unclear how CLL-cell integrins are activated for adhesion to, or movement on, the various adhesive proteins present in lymphoreticular tissues.

In conclusion, SDF-1 and CCR7 ligands, and IL-8 and other chemokines and their receptors, together with α_4 engagement and exposure to HA are all known to have functional effects relevant to homing. However, it is still not possible to give anything like a complete overall picture of the mechanisms involved in malignant cell homing in the disease. This is hardly surprising given that relatively little is known about the mechanisms involved in the homing of memory cells—the presumed normal counterpart of CLL cells.

Proliferation and rescue of CLL cells within tissues

Within tissues, CLL cells are present in so-called proliferation centres or in more or less diffuse infiltrates. The centres of proliferation have a pseudo-follicular structure that lack clearly defined anatomical zones of true follicles, although they do contain dendritic-like cells and T-cells, in addition to the proliferating CLL cells (Vega *et al.* 2002). Thus, within pseudo-follicles, these accessory cells are likely to provide stimuli for both CLL-cell proliferation and protection from apoptosis. Survival of the infiltrating cells outside the proliferation centres involves their interactions with other stromal elements (Lagneaux *et al.* 1999; Granziero *et al* , 2003), including so-called 'nurse cells' (Tsukada *et al.* 2001) and possibly also extracellular matrix components (de la Fuente *et al.* 1999). The adhesion receptors involved in the latter interactions could themselves generate survival signals and/or stimulate production of protective autocrine cytokines.

Indeed, several such autocrine cytokines with a potenial role in CLL-cell rescue from apoptosis have been identified. These include autocrine CXC-type chemokine IL-8 (di Celle *et al.* 1996), ligands for TNF-R superfamily (TNFα and BLyS) (Novak *et al.* 2002) and growth-factors that stimulate either receptor tyrosine-kinases (VEGF and FGF) (Chen *et al.* 2000; Kay *et al.* 2002) or haematopoietic growth-factor receptors (G-CSF) (Corcione & Pistoia 1997). The association of increased plasma levels of some of these growth factors with advanced disease (as defined by the extent of organ involvement) suggests that they may indeed be principally produced by cells within infiltrated tissues and that, at some level of production, these factors may play a role in promoting the survival of both tissue-infiltrating, as well as circulating, CLL cells.

The above survival-promoting autocrine factors can, of course, be derived also from paracrine sources, and by no means exhaust the list of the biological-response modifiers that have been implicated in the pathogenesis of CLL (Orsini *et al.* 2000). Since the majority of such modifiers are immuno-regulatory cytokines, their role in CLL can be best understood in the context of the deregulation of the immune system observed in this disease.

Role of cytokines in the deregulation of immune responses

In CLL, the functional responses of T cells, normal B cells and dendritic cells are often so deregulated that this results in both a general immunodeficiency and a tendency to autoimmunity. This can be at least partly explained by effects that the vastly expanded malignant-cell clone exerts on other cells, either through direct cell-cell contacts or through production or consumption of cytokines.

Historically, the first immunoregulatory cytokine studied in depth in CLL was IL-2. CLL cells express a functional IL-2 receptor that contributes signals for growth and/or differentiation when cells are stimulated with IL-2 in combination with CD-40L, CpG oligonucleotides and/or IL-10 (Decker *et al.* 2000; Tangye *et al.* 2003). IL-2 is produced by T-cells and is mandatory for their growth and it has been suggested that the T-cell abnormalities in CLL result, at least in part from consumption of IL-2 by CLL cells (Burton & Kay 1994).

IL-4 is a TH-2 cytokine first identified as a B-cell growth factor capable of enhancing cell proliferation in response to BCR stimulation. Its role in CLL is suggested by a similar proliferative effect on the malignant cells cultured in the presence of CD40L (Grdisa 2003). IL-4 can also be autocrinely produced by CLL cells (Kay *et al.* 2001) and can protect them from apoptosis by maintaining Bcl-2 expression (Dancescu *et al.* 1992).

IL-6 is a pleiotropic cytokine produced by a variety of cell types, including normal and malignant B cells. This cytokine plays an important role in terminal differentiation of B cells into antibody-secreting cells, and is critical for the development of plasma-cell neoplasias (Lai *et al.* 2002). In CLL, serum levels of both IL-6 and soluble IL-6 receptor are elevated and positively correlate with the severity of the disease (Robak *et al.* 1999). This is particularly evident in patients with autoimmune complications of the disease (Lahat *et al.* 1991). *In vivo* stimulation of malignant CLL cells by IL-6 is suggested by 'constitutive' phosphorylation of STAT3 in these cells (Frank *et al.* 1997; Hirano *et al.* 2000).

IL-10 was first named 'cytokine-synthesis-inhibitory factor' (CSIF) because it inhibits synthesis of TH-1 cytokines including TNFα, IFNγ and IL-1 (Conti *et al.* 2003). The major source of IL-10 are macrophages stimulated through Toll-like receptors (Byrne & Reen 2002). IL-10 suppresses IL-6 production but, in combination with CD40L and IL-2, stimulates differentiation of memory cells into plasma cells. Like IL-6, IL-10 also signals through STAT3, but the signalling by the two cytokines is differentially inhibited by SOCSs (suppressors of cytokine signalling) (Niemand *et al.* 2003). CLL cells produce IL-10 (Fayad *et al.* 2001), but studies of the relationship between IL-10 levels and disease severity and prognosis have given results that vary from showing a positive correlation to absent or inverse associations. This suggests a heterogeneity of CLL in terms of balance between TH1 and TH2 cytokine production where IL-10 plays a key regulatory role.

Summary

This review has addressed the possible origin of CLL and the factors which govern disease progression and prognosis. The phenotype and genotype of CLL-cell clones suggest that they originate from innate-immunity memory cells which are activated to a variable degree, but never fully differentiate into antibody-secreting cells.

The specificity and functional properties of the BCR of the malignant cells suggest that the pathogenesis of CLL may be similar to that of autoimmune disorders such as rheumatoid arthritis (RA) or systemic lupus erythematosis (SLE). The principal difference between CLL and these diseases could all be the consequence of the failure of CLL cells to undergo terminal differentiation into plasma cells and thus to produce antibodies that could clear/neutralise the antigen. The chronic antigenic exposure could then provide stimuli for both slow proliferation and prolonged survival of the malignant cells. The resulting clonal expansion is clearly influenced by a number of intrinsic and extrinsic factors which differ from clone to clone, leading to the pronounced heterogeneity that is likely to influence disease progression. Intrinsic factors identified so far include V_H mutation, Zap-70 expression, BCR responsiveness, p53/ ATM inactivation, CD38 expression and a phenotype that favours tissue infiltration. Among candidate extrinsic factors are antigen drive, TH_2 cytokine predominance and interaction with accessory cells and extracellular matrix. Although several of these intrinsic and extrinsic factors have been associated with the two prognostic groups defined by the extent of somatic V_H mutation, other factors seem more related to the severity of the disease at the time of study, and their prognostic relevance still remains to be established.

References

Albesiano, E., Messmer, B. T., Damle, R. N., Allen, S. L., Rai, K. R. & Chiorazzi, N. (2003). Activation-induced cytidine deaminase in chronic lymphocytic leukemia B cells: expression as multiple forms in a dynamic, variably sized fraction of the clone. *Blood* **102**, 3333–3339.

Allsup, D. J. & Lin, K. *et al.* (2002). Antigen receptor non-responsiveness in chronic lymphocytic leukaemia. *British Journal of Haematology* **117** (Suppl. 1), 208 (abstract).

Balint, E. E. & Vousden, K. H. (2001). Activation and activities of the p53 tumour suppressor protein. *British Journal of Cancer* **85**, 1813–1823.

Bendelac, A., Bonneville, M., Kearney, J. F. (2001). Autoreactivity by design: innate B and T lymphocytes. *Nature Reviews Immunology* **1**, 177–186.

Bernal, A., Pastore, R. D. *et al.* (2001). Survival of leukemic B cells promoted by engagement of the antigen receptor. *Blood* **98**, 3050–3057.

Bohnhorst, J. O., Bjorgan, M. B., Thoen, J. E., Natvig, J. B. & Thompson, K. M. (2001). Bm1–Bm5 classification of peripheral blood B cells reveals circulating germinal center founder cells in healthy individuals and disturbance in the B cell populations in patients with primary Sjogren's syndrome. *Journal of Immunology* **167**, 3610–3618.

Bullrich, F., Rasio, D., Kitada, S., Starostik, P., Kipps, T., Keating, M., Albitar, M., Reed, J. C. & Croce, C. M. (1999). ATM mutations in B-cell chronic lymphocytic leukemia. *Cancer Research* **59**, 24–27.

Burger, J. A., Burger, M. & Kipps, T. J. (1999). Chronic lymphocytic leukemia B cells express functional CDCR4 chemokine receptors that mediate spontaneous migration beneath bone marrow stromal cells. *Blood* **94**, 3658–3667.

Burton, J. & Kay, N. E. (1994). Does IL-2 receptor expression and secretion in chronic B-cell leukemia have a role in down-regulation of the immune system? *Leukemia* **8**, 92–96.

Byrne, A. & Reen, D. J. (2002). Lipopolysaccharide induces rapid production of IL-10 by monocytes in the presence of apoptotic neutrophils. *Journal of Immunology* **168**, 1968–1977.

Cantwell, M. & Hua, T. *et al.* (1997). Acquired CD40-ligand deficiency in chronic lymphocytic leukemia. *Nature Medicine* **3**, 984–989.

Cerutti, A., Kim, E. C. *et al.* (2001). Dysregulation of CD30+ T cells by leukemia impairs isotype switching in normal B cells. *Nature Immunology* **2**, 150–156.

Chen, H., Treweeke, A. T. *et al.* (2000). In vitro and in vivo production of vascular endothelial growth factor by chronic lymphocytic leukaemia cells. *Blood* **96**, 3181–3187.

Chen, J. R., Gu, B. J. *et al.* (1999). Transendothelial migration of lymphocytes in chronic lymphocytic leukaemia is impaired and involves down-regulation of both L-selectin and CD23. *British Journal of Haematology* **105**, 181–189.

Chen, L., Widhopf, G., Huynh, L., Rassenti, L., Rai, K. R., Weiss, A. & Kipps, T. J. (2002). Expression of ZAP-70 is associated with increased B-cell receptor signalling in chronic lymphocytic leukemia. *Blood* **100**, 4609–4614.

Chiorazzi, N. & Ferrarini, M. (2003). B cell chronic lymphocytic leukemia: lessons learned from studies of the B cell antigen receptor. *Annual Review of Immunology* **21**, 841–894.

Conti, P, Kempuraj, D. *et al.* (2003). IL-10, an inflammatory/inhibitory cytokine, but not always. *Immunology Letters* **86**, 123–129.

Corcione, A. & Pistoia, V. (1997). B-cell-derived granulocyte-colony stimulating factor (G-CSF). *Elsevier: Methods* **11**, 143–147.

Cordone, I., Masi, S., Mauro, F. R., Soddu, S., Morsilli, O., Valentini, T., Vegna, M. L., Guglielmi, C., Mancini, F., Giuliacci, S., Sacchi, A., Mandelli, F. & Foa, R. (1998). p53 expression in B-cell chronic lymphocytic leukemia: a marker of disease progression and poor prognosis. *Blood* **91**,4342–4349.

Crespo, M., Bosch, F., Villamor, N., Bellosillo, B., Colomer, D., Rozman, M., Marce, S., Lopez-Guillermo, A., Campo, E. & Montserrat, E. (2003). ZAP-70 expression as a surrogate for immunoglobulin-variable-region mutations in chronic lymphocytic leukemia. *New England Journal of Medicine* **348**,1764–1775.

Damle, R. N., Wasil, T. *et al.* (1999). IgV gene mutation status and CD38 expression as novel prognostic indicators in chronic lymphocytic leukaemia. *Blood* **94**, 1840–1847.

Damle, R. N., Ghiotto, F. *et al.* (2002). B-cell chronic lymphocytic leukemia cells express a surface membrane phenotype of activated, antigen-experienced B lymphocytes. *Blood* **99**, 4087–4093.

Dammers, P. M., Visser, A., Popa, E. R., Nieuwenhuis, P. & Kroese, F. G. M. (2000). Most marginal zone B cells in rat express germline encoded Ig V_H genes and are ligand selected. *Journal of Immunology* **165**, 6156–6169.

Dancescu, M., Rubio-Trujillo, M. *et al.* (1992). Interleukin 4 protects chronic lymphocytic leukemic B cells from death by apoptosis and upregulates Bcl-2 expression. *Journal of Experimental Medicine* **176**, 1319–1326.

Dazzi, F., D'Andrea, E. *et al.* (1995). Failure of B cells of chronic lymphocytic leukemia in presenting soluble and allo-antigens. *Clinical Immunology and Immunopathology* **75**, 26–32.

Deaglio, S., Mallone, R. *et al* (2000). CD38/CD31, a receptor ligand system ruling adhesion and signalling in human lymphocytes. *Chemical Immunology* **75**, 99–120.

Deaglio, S., Capobianco, A. *et al.* (2003). CD38 is a signalling molecule in B-cell chronic lymphocytic leukaemia cells. *Blood* **102**, 2146–2155.

Decker, T., Schneller, F. *et al.* (2000). Immunostimulatory CpG-oligonucleotides induce functional high affinity IL-2 receptors on B-CLL cells: costimulation with IL-2 results in a highly immunogenic phenotype. *Experimental Hematology* **28**, 558–568.

de la Fuente, M. T., Casanova B. *et al.* (1999). Fibronectin interaction with alpha4beta1 integrin prevents apoptosis in B cell chronic lymphocytic leukemia: correlation with Bcl-2 and Bax. *Leukemia* **13**, 266–274.

de Vinuesa, C. G., Cook, M. C. *et al* (2000). Germinal centers without T cells. *Journal of Experimental Medicine* **191**, 485–493.

di Celle, P., Mariani, S. *et al.* (1996). Interleukin-8 induces the accumulation of B-cell chronic lymphocytic leukemia cells by prolonging survival in an autocrine fashion. *Blood* **87**, 4382–4389.

Dohner, H., Fischer, C., Bentz, M., Hansen, K., Benner, A., Cabot, G., Diehl, D., Schlenk, R., Coy, J., Stilgenbauer, S., Volkmann, M., Galle, P.R., Poustka, A., Hunstein, W. & Lichter, P. (1995). p53 gene deletion predicts for poor survival and non-response to therapy with purine analogues in chronic B-cell leukaemias. *Blood* **85**, 1580–1589.

Dohner, H., Stilgenbauer, S., Benner, A., Leupolt, E., Krober, A., Bullinger, L., Dohner, K., Bentz, M. & Lichter, P. (2000). Genomic aberrations and survival in chronic lymphocytic leukemia. *New England Journal of Medicine* **343**, 1910–1916.

El Rouby, S., Thomas, A., Costin, D., Rosenberg, C.R., Potmesil, M., Silber, R. & Newcombe, E. W. (1993). p53 gene mutation in B-cell chronic lymphocytic leukemia is associated with drug resistance and is independent of MDR1/MDR3 gene expression. *Blood* **82**, 3452–3459.

Euler, W. J., Christensen, S. & Shlomchik, M. J. (2002). Evolution of autoantibody responses via somatic hypermutation outside of germinal centers. *Science* **297**, 2006–2008.

Fagnoni, F. F., Vescovini, R. *et al.* (2000). Shortage of circulating naïve CD8(+) T cells provides new insights on immunodeficiency in aging. *Blood* **95**, 2860–2868.

Fais, F., Ghiotto, F. *et al.* (1998). Chronic lymphocytic leukemia B cells express restricted sets of mutated and unmutated antigen receptors. *Journal of Clinical Investigation* **102**, 1515–1525.

Fayad, L., Keating, M. J. *et al.* (2001). Interleukin-6 and interleukin-10 levels in chronic lymphocytic leukemia: correlation with phenotypic characteristics and outcome. *Blood* **97**, 256–263.

Fillatreau, S., Sweenie, C. H. *et al.* (2002). B cells regulate autoimmunity by provision of IL-10. *Nature Immunology* **3**, 944–950.

Frank, D. A., Mahajan, S. & Ritz, J. (1997). B lymphocytes from patients with chronic lymphocytic leukemia contain signal transducer and activator of transcription (STAT) 1 and STAT3 constitutively phosphorylated on serine residues. *Journal of Clinical Investigation* **100**, 3140–3148.

Furman, R. R., Asgary, Z. et al. (2000). Modulation of NF-kappa B activity and apoptosis in chronic lymphocytic leukemia B cells. *Journal of Immunology* **164**, 2200–2206.

Ghia, P., Guida, G. et al (2003). The pattern of CD38 defines a distinct subset of chronic lymphocytic leukemia (CLL) patients at risk of disease progression. *Blood* **101**, 162–169.

Granziero, L., Circosta, P. et al. (2003). CD100/Plexin-B1 interactions sustain proliferation and survival of normal and leukemic CD5+ B lymphocytes. *Blood* **101**, 1962–1969.

Grdisa, M. (2003). Influence of CD40 ligation on survival and apoptosis of B-CLL cells in vitro. *Leukemia Research* **27**, 951–956.

Hamblin, T. J., Davis. Z. et al. (1999). Unmutated IgV(H) genes are associated with a more aggressive form of chronic lymphocytic leukaemia. *Blood* **94**,1848–1854.

He, X., Goronzy, J. J. et al. (1995). VH3-21 B cells escape from a state of tolerance in rheumatoid arthritis and secrete rheumatoid factor. *Molecular Medicine* **1**, 768–780.

Hirano, T., Ishihara, K. & Hibi, M. (2000). Roles of STAT3 in mediating the cell growth, differentiation, and survival signals relayed through the IL-6 family of cytokine reeptors. *Oncogene* **19**, 2548–2556.

Huber, S. A., Kupperman, J. & Newell, M. K. (1999). Hormonal regulation of CD4 + T cell responses in coxsackievirus B3-induced myocarditis in mice. *Journal of Virology* **73**, 4689–4695.

Ibrahim, S., Keating, M. et al. (2001). CD38 expression is an important prognostic factor in B-cell chronic lymphocytic leukemia. *Blood* **98**, 181–186.

Johnson, S. A., Rozzo, S. J. & Cambier, J. C. (2002). Aging-dependent exclusion of antigen-inexperienced cells from the peripheral B cell repertoire. *Journal of Immunology* **168**, 5014–5023.

Jones, D., Benjamin, R. J., Shatisafaei, A. & Dorfman, D. M. (2000). The chemokine receptor CXCR3 is expressed in a subset of B-cell lymphomas and is a marker of B chronic lymphocytic leukemia. *Blood* **95**, 27–632.

Kay, N. E., Han, L., Bone, N. & Williams, G. (2001). Interleukin 4 content in chronic lymphocytic leukaemia (CLL) B cells and blood CD8+ T cells from B-CLL patients: impact on clonal B-cell apoptosis. *British Journal of Haematology* **112**, 760–767.

Kay, N. E., Bone, N. D. et al. (2002). B-CLL cells are capable of synthesis and secetion of both pro- and anti-angiogenic molecules. *Leukemia* **16**, 911–919.

Kay, N. E., Hamblin, T. J., Jelinek, D. F., Dewald, G. W., Byrd, J. C., Farag, S., Lucas, M. & Lin, T. (2002). Chronic lymphocytic leukemia. *Hematology (American Society of Hematology Educational Program)*, 193–213.

Klein, U., Kuppers, R. & Rajewsky, K. (1997). Evidence for a large compartment of IgM-expressing memory B cells in humans. *Blood* **89**, 1288–1298.

Klein, U., Tu, Y., Stolovitzky, G. A. et al. (2001). Gene expression profiling of B cell chronic lymphocytic leukemia reveals a homogeneous phenotype related to memory B cells. *Journal of Experimental Medicine* **194**, 1625–1638.

Konoplera, M., Rissling, I. & Andreeff, M. (2000). CD38 in hematopoietic malignancies. In *Human CD38 and related molecules* (ed. K. Melita & F. Malavasi) (*Chemical Immunology* **75**), pp. 189–206. Basel: Karger.

Kröber, A., Buhler, A. et al. (2001). Analysis of VDJ rearrangement structure and VH mutation status in chronic lymphocytic leukemia. *Blood* **98**, 358a (abstract).

Kröber, A., Seiler, T. *et al*. (2002a). V(H) mutation status, CD38 expression level, genomic aberrations, and survival in chronic lymphocytic leukemia. *Blood* **100**,1410–1416.

Kröber, A., Benner, A. *et al*. (2002b). Multivariate analysis of specific VH-genes in CLL: V3-21 and V3-23 are prognostic factors independent of the VH mutation status. *Blood* **100**, 196a (abstract).

Lagneaux, L., Delforge, A. *et al*. (1999). Adhesion to bone marrow stroma inhibits apoptosis of chronic lymphocytic leukemia cells. *Leukemia & Lymphoma* **35**, 445–453.

Lahat, N., Aghai, E. *et al*. (1991). Increased spontaneous secretion of IL-6 from B cells of patients with B-chronic lymphatic leukaemia (B-CLL) and autoimmunity. *Clinical and Experimental Immunology* **85**, 302–306.

Lai, R., O'Brien, S. *et al*. (2002). Prognostic value of plasma interleukin-6 levels in patients with chronic lymphocytic leukemia. *Cancer* **95**, 1071–1075.

Lane, D. P. (1992). p53, guardian of the genome. *Nature* **358**, 15–16.

Lanham, S., Hamblin T. *et al*. (2003). Differential signalling via surface IgM is associated with VH gene mutational status and CD38 expression in chronic lymphocytic leukemia. *Blood* **101**, 1087–1093.

Lens, D., Dyer, M. J., Garcia-Marco, J.M., De Schouwer, P.J., Hamoudi, R.A., Jones, D., Farahat, N., Matutes, E. & Catovsky, D. (1997). p53 abnormalities in CLL are associated with excess of prolymphocytes and poor prognosis. *British Journal of Haematology* **99**, 848–857.

Lin, K., Manocha, S. *et al*. (2003). High frequency of p53 dysfunction and low level of V_H mutation in chronic lymphocytic leukemia patients using the V_H3-21 gene segment. *Blood* **102**, 1145–1146.

Lin, K., Sherrington, P. D. *et al*. (2002). Relationship between p53 dysfunction, CD38 expression, and IgV(H) mutation in chronic lymphocytic leukemia. *Blood* **100**, 1404–1409.

Lucas, A. H., Moulton, K. D., Tang, V. R. & Reason, D. C. (2001). Combinational library cloning of human antibodies to *streptococcus pneumoniae* capsular polysaccharides: variable region primary structures and evidence for somatic mutation of Fab fragments specific for capsular serotypes 6B, 14, and 213F. *Infection and Immunity* **69**, 853–864.

Marchalonis, J. J., Kaveri, S. *et al*. (2002). Natural recognition repertoire and the evolutionary emergence of the combinatorial immune system. *FASEB Journal* **16**, 842–848.

Martin, F. & Kearney, J. F. (2000). B-cell subsets and the mature preimmune repertoire. Marginal zone and B1 B cells as part of a "natural immune memory". *Immunological Reviews* **175**, 70–79.

Martin, F., Oliver, A. M. & Kearney, J. F. (2001). Marginal zone and B1 B cells unite in the early response against T-independent blood-borne particulate antigens. *Immunity* **14**, 617–629.

Matrai, Z., Lin, K. *et al*. (2001). CD38 expression and IgVH gene mutation B-cell chronic lymphocytic leukemia. *Blood* **97**, 1902–1903.

McCarthy, H., Wierda, W. G., Barron, L. L., Cromwell, C. C., Wang, J., Coombes, K. R., Rangel, R., Elenitoba-Johnson, K. S., Keating, M. J. & Abruzzo, L. V. (2003). High expression of activation-induced cytidine deaminase (AID) and splice variants is a distinctive feature of poor-prognosis chronic lymphocytic leukemia. *Blood* **101**, 4903–4908.

Naylor, M. & Capra, J. D. (1999). Mutational status of Ig V_H genes provides clinically valuable information in B-cell chronic lymphocytic leukaemia. *Blood* **94**, 1837–1839.

Newkirk, M. M. (2002). Rheumatoid factors: host resistance or autoimmunity? *Clinical Immunology* **104**, 1–13.

Niemand, C., Nimmesgern, A. *et al.* (2003). Activation of STAT3 by IL-6 and IL-10 in primary human macrophages is differentially modulated by suppressor of cytokine signalling. *Journal of Immunology* **170**, 3263–3272.

Nollet, F., Cauwelier, B. *et al.* (2002). Do B-cell chronic lymphocytic leukemia patients with Ig VH3-21 genes constitute a new subset of chronic lymphocytic leukemia? *Blood* **100**, 1097–1098.

Novak, A. J., Bram, R. J. *et al.* (2002). Aberrant expression of B-lymphocyte stimulator by B chronic lymphocytic leukemia cells: a mechanism for survival. *Blood* **100**, 2973–2979.

Orchard, J. A., Ibbotson, R. E., Davis, Z., Wiestner, A., Rosenwald, A., Thomas, P. W., Hamblin, T. J., Staudt, L. M., Oscier, D. G. (2004). ZAP-70 expression and prognosis in chronic lymphocytic leukaemia. *The Lancet* **363**, 105–111.

Orsini, E., Guarini, A. & Foa, R. (2000). Accessory cells, cytokine loops and cell-to-cell interactions in chronic lymphocytic leukemia. *Reviews in Clinical Experimental Hematology* **4**, 73–98.

Orsini, E., Guarini, A. *et al.* (2003). The circulating dendritic cell compartment in patients with chronic lymphocytic leukemia is severely defective and unable to stimulate an effective T-cell response. *Cancer Research* **63**, 4497–4506.

Oscier, D. G., Gardiner, A. C. *et al.* (2002). Multivariate analysis of prognostic factors in CLL: clinical stage, VH gene mutational status, and loss or mutation of the p53 gene are independent prognostic factors. *Blood* **100**, 1177–1184.

Partida-Sanchez, S., Cockayne, D. A. *et al.* (2001). Cyclic ADP-ribose production by CD38 regulates intracellular calcium release, extracellular calcium influx and chemotaxis in neutrophils and is required for bacterial clearance *in vivo*. *Nature Medicine* **7**, 1209–1216.

Pettitt, A. R., Sherrington, P. D., Stewart, G., Cawley, J. C., Taylor, A. M. & Stankovic, T. (2001). p53 dysfunction in B-cell chronic lymphocytic leukemia: inactivation of ATM as an alternative to TP53 mutation. *Blood* **98**, 814–822.

Potter, K. N., Orchard, J. *et al.* (2003). Features of the overexpressed V1-69 genes in the unmutated subset of chronic lymphocytice leukemia are distinct from those in the healthy elderly repertoire. *Blood* **101**, 3082–3084.

Pritsch, O., Magnac, C. *et al.* (1993). V gene usage by seven hybrids derived from CD5+ B-cell chronic lymphocytic leukemia and displaying autoantibody activity. *Blood* **82**, 3103–3112.

Robak, T., Wierzbowska, A. *et al.* (1999). Serum levels of IL-6 type cytokines and soluble IL-6 receptors in active B-cell chronic lymphocytic leukemia and in cladribine induced remission. *Mediators of Inflammation* **8**, 277–286.

Rosenwald, A., Alizadeh, A. A. *et al.* (2001). Relation of gene expression phenotype to immunoglobulin mutation genotype in B cell chronic lymphocytic leukemia. *Journal of Experimental Medicine* **194**, 1639–1647.

Sallusto, F., MacKay, C. R. & Lanzavecchia, A. (2000). The role of chemokine receptors in primary, effector and memory immune responses. *Annual Reviews of Immunology* **18**, 393–620.

Schuler, M., Tretter, T. *et al.* (1999). Autocrine transforming growth factor-beta from chronic lymphocytic leukemia-B cells interferes with proliferative T cell signals. *Immunobiology* **200**, 128–139.

Scrivener, S., Goddard, R. V. *et al.* (2003). Abnormal T-cell function in B-cell chronic lymphocytic leukaemia. *Leukemia & Lymphoma* **44**, 383–389.

Shi, Y., Agematsu, K., Ochs, H. D. & Sugane, K. (2003). Functional analysis of human memory B-cell subpopulations: IgD+CD27+ B cells are crucial in secondary immune response by producing high affinity IgM. *Clinical Immunology* **108**, 128–137.

Shokri, F., Mageed, R.A., Richardson, P. & Jefferis, R. (1993). Modulation and high frequency expression of autoantibody-associated cross-reactive idiotypes linked to the VHI subgroup in CD5-expressing B lymphocytes from patients with chronic lymphocytic leukaemia (B-CLL). *Scandinavian Journal of Immunology* **37**, 673–679.

Stankovic, T., Stewart, G. S., Byrd, P., Fegan, C., Moss, P. A. & Taylor, A. M. (2002a). ATM mutations in sporadic lymphoid tumours. *Leukemia & Lymphoma* **43**, 1563–1571.

Stankovic, T., Stewart, G. S., Fegan, C., Biggs, P., Last, J., Byrd, P. J., Keenan, R. D., Moss, P. A., Taylor, A. M. (2002b). Ataxia telangiectasia mutated-deficient B-cell chronic lymphocytic leukemia occurs in pregerminal center cells and results in defective damage response and unrepaired chromosome damage. *Blood* **99**, 300–309.

Stankovic, T., Weber, P., Stewart, G., Bedenham, T., Murray, J., Byrd, P. J., Moss, P. A. & Taylor, A. M. (1999). Inactivation of ataxia telangiectasia mutated gene in B-cell chronic lymphocytic leukaemia. *The Lancet* **353**, 26–29.

Starostik, P., Manshouri, T., O'Brien, S., Freireich, E., Kantarjian, H., Haidar, M., Lerner, S., Keating, M. & Albitar, M. (1998). Deficiency of the ATM protein expression defines an aggressive subgroup of B-cell chronic lymphocytic leukemia. *Cancer Research* **58**, 4552–4557.

Tangye, S. G., Avery, D. T., Deenick, E. K. & Hodgkin, P. D. (2003). Intrinsic differences in the proliferation of the naïve and memory human B cells as a mechanism for enhanced secondary immune responses. *Journal of Immunology* **170**, 686–694.

Till, K. J., Zuzel, M. & Cawley, J. C. (1999). The role of hyaluronan and IL-8 in the migration of chronic lymphocytic leukemia cells within lymphoreticular tissues. *Cancer Research* **59**, 4419–4426.

Till, K. J., Lin, K., Zuzel, M. & Cawley, J. C. (2001). The chemokine receptor CCR7 and α4 integrin are important for migration of chronic lymphocytic leukemia cells into lymph nodes. *Blood* **99**, 2977–2984.

Tobin, G., Thunberg, U. *et al.* (2002). Somatically mutated Ig V(H)3-21 genes characterize a new subset of chronic lymphocytic leukemia. *Blood* **99**, 2262–2264.

Tobin, G., Thunberg, U., Johnson, A., Eriksson, I., Soderberg, O., Karlsson, K., Merup, M., Juliusson, G., Vilpo, J., Enblad, G., Sundstrom, C., Roos, G. & Rosenquisr, R. (2003). Chronic lymphocytic leukemias utilizing the VH3-21 gene display highly restricted Vlambda2-14 gene usage and homologous CDR3s: implicating recognition of a common antigen epitope. *Blood* **101**, 4952–4957.

Tsukada, N., Burger, J. A., Zvaifler, N. J. & Kipps, T. J. (2002). Distinctive features of "nurselike" cells that differentiate in the context of chronic lymphocytic leukemia. *Blood* **99**, 1030–1037.

Vega, F., Medeiros, J. *et al.* (2002). The stromal composition of malignant lymphoid aggregates in bone marrow: variations in architecture and phenotype in different B-cell tumours. *British Journal of Haematology* **117**, 569–576.

Vincent, A., Cawley, J. C. & Burthem, J. (1996). Integrin function in chronic lymphocytic leukemia. *Blood* **87**, 4780–4788.

Vogelstein, B., Lane, D. & Levine, A. J. (2000). Surfing the p53 network. *Nature* **408**, 307–310.

Wattel, E., Preudhomme, C., Hecquet, B., Vanrumbeke, M., Quesnel, B., Dervite, E., Morel, P. & Fenaux, P. (1994). p53 mutations are associated with resistance to chemotherapy and short survival in hematologic malignancies. *Blood* **84**, 3148–3157.

Weller, S., Faili, A., Garcia, C., Braun, M. C., Le Deist, F. F., de Saint Basile, G. G., Hermine, O., Fischer, A., Reynaud, C. A. & Weill, J. C. (2001). CD40–CD40L independent Ig gene hypermutation suggests a second B cell diversification pathway in humans. *Proceedings of the National Academy of Sciences of the United States of America* **98**, 1166–1170.

Wierda, W. G., Cantwell, M. J., Woods, S. J., Rassenti, L. Z., Prussak, C. E. & Kipps, T. J. (2000). CD40-ligand (CD154) gene therapy for chronic lymphocytic leukemia. *Blood* **96**, 2917–2924.

Wiestner, A., Rosenwald, A., Barry, T. S., Wright, G., Davis, R. E., Henrickson, S. E., Zhao, H., Ibbotson, R. E., Orchard, J. A., Davis, Z., Stetler-Stevenson, M., Raffeld, M., Arthur, D. C., Marti, G. E., Wilson, W. H., Hamblin, T. J., Oscier, D. G., Staudt, L. M. (2003). ZAP-70 expression identifies a chronic lymphocytic leukemia subtype with unmutated immunoglobulin genes, inferior clinical outcome, and distinct gene expression profile. *Blood* **101**, 4944–4951.

Wilder, R. L. (1998). Hormones, pregnancy and autoimmune diseases. *Annals of the New York Academy of Science* **840**, 45–50.

Worthylake, R. A. & Burridge, K. (2001). Leukocyte transendothelial migration: orchestrating the underlying molecular machinery. *Current Opinions in Cell Biology* **13**, 569–577.

Xiaoli, L., Martin, F. *et al.* (2001). Antigen receptor proximal signalling in splenic B-2 cell subsets. *Journal of Immunology* **166**, 3122–3129.

Zupo, S., Isnardi, L. *et al.* (1996). CD38 expression distinguishes two groups of B-cell chronic lymphocytic leukaemias with different responses to anti-IgM antibodies and propensity to apoptosis. *Blood* **88**, 1365–1374.

Zupo, S., Massara, R. *et al.* (2000). Apoptosis or plasma cell differentiation of CD38-positive B-cell chronic lymphocytic leukemia induced by cross-linking of surface IgM or IgD. *Blood* **95**, 1199–1206.

PART 2

Evidence and opinion for medical intervention – I

Chapter 4

Diagnosis and classification of chronic lymphocytic leukaemia

Estella Matutes

Introduction

Chronic lymphocytic leukaemia (CLL) is the most common type of leukaemia in the Western World. It affects adults (65–75 years of age), but is rare below 40 years. The initial clinical manifestations and the disease course are very heterogeneous. Whereas some patients are asymptomatic and the disease is discovered on a routine check-up, others present with widespread and progressive disease.

Regardless of earlier definitions used by the International Workshop on Chronic Lymphocytic Leukaemia (IWCLL) and the National Cancer Institute (NCI), a diagnosis of CLL should be considered in patients with lymphocytosis greater than $3 \times 10^9/l$ with circulating mature-looking lymphocytes (Oscier *et al.* 2004). Demonstration of B-cell clonality in cases with mild lymphocytosis is a useful and key test to confirm the diagnosis of CLL and rule out reactive conditions. A threshold of 30% or more lymphocytes in the bone marrow aspirate is also used as a diagnostic criterion.

Cell morphology and immunophenotype are the two key laboratory tests to establish the diagnosis of CLL. They are simple and easy to perform in routine practice and, in most cases, allow distinction of CLL from other primary leukaemias and lymphomas in the leukaemic phase. In a few cases who present diagnostic difficulties, information is needed from other investigations, such as tissue histology and molecular genetics, to establish the diagnosis with certainty. The latter test is not only helpful as a diagnostic tool but also provides relevant prognostic information.

Here I describe the morphological features and immunophenotypical profile of chronic lymphocytic leukaemia (CLL) and discuss the value of these investigations as front-line diagnostic tests. I emphasise too their correlation with the clinical features, disease progression and molecular genetics.

Morphology

The cell morphology described by the French–American–British (FAB) group (Bennett *et al.* 1989) provides useful information to distinguish CLL from other lymphoproliferative disorders. The cytological features are best appreciated in well-stained and freshly prepared peripheral blood films rather than in bone marrow smears and/or tissue imprints. Still, as there may be variation in morphology among tissues, e.g. the presence of large cells in one and not in another, analysis of specimens other than peripheral blood is recommended. According to the lymphocyte morphology of the circulating cells, two groups of CLL are distinguished (Matutes *et al.* 1996; Matutes and Polliack 2000), which are as follows.

(a) Typical CLL

This is the most common form, accounting for 80–85% of cases. Most (>90%) cells are small to medium size, with scant cytoplasm and regular nuclear outline with clumped chromatin; nucleoli, if present, are inconspicuous (Figure 4.1). A small proportion of cells may be larger, with prolymphocytoid features or have an indented or irregular nucleus, but they account for fewer than 10% of cells. A typical feature of CLL is the presence of smudge (basket) cells on the smears, the so-called Gumprecht phenomenon.

(b) Atypical CLL

This group represents around 15% of CLL cases and comprises two subtypes (Matutes *et al.* 1996; Matutes and Polliack 2000): (i) CLL with increased (>10%) prolymphocytes designated CLL/PL; (ii) 'atypical' CLL with lymphoplasmacytic features and/or cleaved cells, designated by the FAB group mixed-cell type (Bennett *et al.* 1989).

CLL/PL was already recognised in the late 1970s as a distinct form of CLL and described as 'prolymphocytoid' transformation of CLL. CLL/PL may be apparent at diagnosis or develop during the course of the disease. The morphology of CLL/PL is distinct and characterised by a mixture of typical CLL cells and larger nucleolated prolymphocytoid cells (Figure 4.2); occasional immunoblast cells with abundant basophilic cytoplasm containing one or two nucleoli may also be identified. The criterion to define CLL/PL is the presence of more than 10% prolymphocytoid or 'paraimmunoblast' cells in the peripheral blood. CLL/PL can be considered as a subtle transformation of CLL as patients have clinical features and a disease course intermediate between CLL and B-prolymphocytic leukaemia (B-PLL), e.g. high lymphocyte counts, marked splenomegaly, progressive disease and higher proliferative rate as estimated by Ki-67 expression (Cordone *et al.* 1992).

The second group of CLL with atypical morphology is designated 'atypical' CLL. In these cases there is also a mixture of typical CLL lymphocytes and cells displaying more abundant basophilic cytoplasm and/or cells with an indented or cleaved nucleus (Figure 4.3). The threshold considered for the diagnosis of atypical CLL is the presence of 15% or more circulating atypical cells. Clinical features are similar to those of typical CLL although the disease course may be closer to that of CLL/PL, perhaps underlined by similar cytogenetic/molecular features.

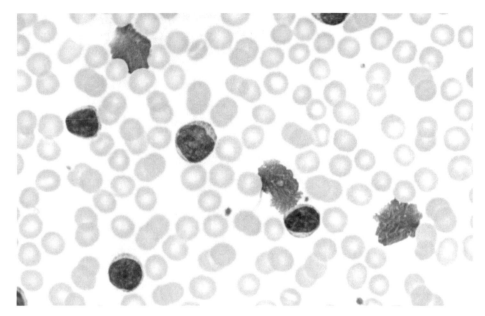

Figure 4.1 Circulating lymphocytes from a typical CLL showing that most cells are small with scanty cytoplasm and clumped nuclear chromatin.

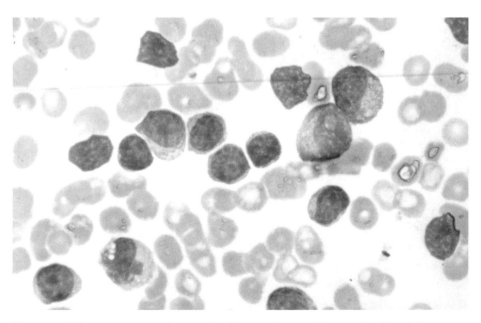

Figure 4.2 Circulating cells from a CLL/PL showing a mixture of cells with features characteristic of CLL and others with larger size, less condensed chromatin and nucleolus (prolymphocytoid cells).

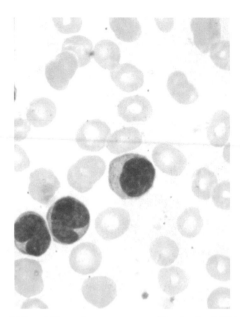

Figure 4.3 Peripheral blood films from a case with atypical CLL, showing lymphocytes with condensed chromatin and a cleaved/indented nucleus.

(c) Richter's syndrome

Although not considered formerly as a morphological group of CLL, it should be noted that Richter's syndrome or transformation of CLL into a large cell lymphoma may involve the blood, or even present with the blood and the marrow as the unique sites of transformation. The peripheral blood film shows the presence of small CLL-like cells and a variable proportion of large cells with reticular chromatin, several nucleoli and abundant basophilic cytoplasm (Figure 4.4). In this context, immunological markers are important in diagnosis as the large cells usually have a phenotype similar to that of CLL cells with minor deviations. As a rule, tumour cells have a high proliferative rate, frequent abnormalities of the p53 tumour suppressor gene; prognosis and outcome are poor.

Table 4.1 shows the correlation between morphology with clinical course and molecular genetics in CLL.

Beyond its diagnostic value, CLL morphology seems to have an impact on disease outcome. A retrospective analysis in over 200 patients has shown that those with atypical CLL and CLL/PL have a significantly higher tendency for progression and treatment need independent of other features such as the presence of trisomy 12 (Oscier *et al.* 1997). Prospective data from the Medical Research Council (MRC) CLL3 trial on more than 600 newly diagnosed CLL patients has established that morphology is a prognostic factor for survival particularly in stage A (Matutes *et al.* 1999a). In addition, the estimate of the proportion of prolymphocytes (more than or

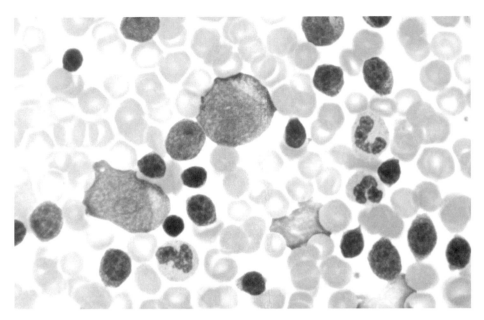

Figure 4.4 Peripheral blood film from a patient with Richter's syndrome showing the presence of very large immunoblasts.

Table 4.1 Correlation between morphology with clinical course and molecular genetics in CLL

Feature	Typical CLL	Atypical CLL*
Clinical course	stable	progressive
Prognosis	good	poor
IgVH	mutated	unmutated
Ki-67	low	higher
CD38	negative	positive
Trisomy 12	rare	frequent
p53 abnormalities	rare	frequent

*Comprises CLL/PL and atypical CLL.

less than 5%) in either typical CLL or CLL/PL had a prognostic impact. Therefore, it is apparent that morphology is an important and easily measurable prognostic factor to predict progression and survival in CLL, particularly in early clinical stages.

An association between morphology and molecular genetics has been documented in CLL. Thus, cases with CLL/PL and atypical CLL more often have trisomy 12 and a higher proliferative rate, whereas 13q14 deletions as a single abnormality in atypical CLL are rare (Matutes *et al.* 1996; Criel *et al.* 1994; Cordone *et al.* 1992). Atypical morphology has been reported in CLL cases with t(14;19) involving the BCL3 gene (Michaux *et al.* 1997). This translocation is exceedingly rare in CLL and it has only been documented in 20 cases. Another infrequent abnormality detected either by cytogenetics or fluorescence *in situ* hybridisation (FISH) is t(11;14) (q13;q32) leading to BCL-1 rearrangement. Most of the cases described are atypical CLL, CLL/PL or CLL with Richter's transformation (Cuneo *et al.* 1995, 1997; Brito-Babapulle *et al.* 1992) and there are uncertainties as to whether most of them would correspond to mantle-cell lymphomas (MCLs) (Matutes *et al.* 1999b). Thus, despite the possibility that the t(11;14) or BCL-1 rearrangement might be a feature in a minority of atypical CLL, in patients with both atypical morphology and immunophenotype (e.g. low CLL scores) the possibility of MCL in leukaemic phase needs to be excluded. It also seems that atypical morphology and CLL/PL are associated with cases that have no mutations (germ-line configuration) of the VH region of the immunoglobulin (Ig) gene, which are shown to have a poorer survival (Hamblin *et al.* 1999).

Immunological markers

Immunophenotyping is a solid benchmark for the diagnosis of CLL, and a mandatory test to be performed in all cases to confirm the diagnosis suspected by morphology and to rule out that of other B- and T-cell disorders. In a broad sense, immunological markers allow us to: (1) distinguish immature or lymphoblastic leukaemias from mature lymphoproliferative disorders; and (2) separate B- from T-cell derived conditions by the expression of surface immunoglobulins (SmIgs) and/or a pan-B cell and T-cell marker (Matutes 1995). Within the B-cell diseases, immunophenotyping also allows us to establish the clonal nature of the disease by showing Ig light-chain restriction, and it provides important diagnostic information by demonstrating profiles typical of certain disorders, in particular for distinguishing CLL from other B-cell malignancies evolving with leukaemia. Documentation of B-cell clonality is important too in differentiating neoplastic B-cell disorders from a rare and benign condition designated polyclonal B-cell lymphocytosis, which is seen preferentially in middle-aged female smokers.

The immunological repertoire of CLL is close to that of a mantle zone lymphocyte present in the secondary reactive follicle centres. Indeed, it has been suggested that CLL arises from a CD5$^+$ mantle-zone lymphocyte that produces autoantibodies (Caligaris-Cappio 1996).

CLL cells have a distinct and unique immunological profile different from that seen in other lymphoid disorders. The typical CLL phenotype is: CD5$^+$, CD23$^+$, FMC7$^-$, weak expression of SmIg and dim or absent expression of membrane CD22 and CD79b. (Figure 4.5). The latter marker identifies an extracellular epitope of the

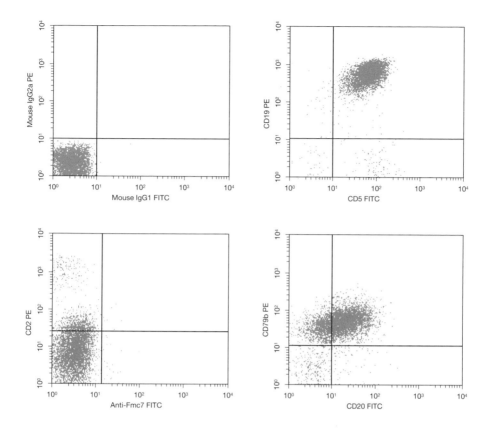

Figure 4.5 Flow cytometry plot of a CLL case showing a characteristic CLL immunophenotype. Most cells are CD5⁺, FMC7⁻ and express weakly CD79b and CD20.

Table 4.2 Scoring system for the diagnosis of CLL

Marker	Points	
	1	0
CD5	positive	negative
CD23	positive	negative
FMC7	negative	positive
SmIg	weak	moderate/strong
CD22/CD79b	weak/negative	moderate/strong

Scores in CLL range from 3 to 5 whereas in the other B-cell disorders they are 0–2 (Matutes *et al.* 1994; Matutes & Polliack 2000).

B-cell receptor beta chain. Its weak or absent expression in CLL might relate to the expression of a truncated form of this molecule and explain the abnormal signal transduction of CLL cells similar to that of anergic B lymphocytes (Thompson *et al.* 1997; Alfarano *et al.* 1999). As no single marker is specific for CLL, a composite phenotype considering this set of five or six markers compounded into a scoring system helps to distinguish CLL from other chronic B-cell malignancies (Matutes *et al.* 1994; Matutes and Polliack, 2000; Matutes 2002) (Table 4.2). Recent studies have shown that the monoclonal antibody (McAb) FMC7 recognises a particular epitope of the multimeric CD20 complex. A few reports have suggested that FMC7 parallels that of CD20 expression in leukaemic CLL cells and thus the latter McAb could replace FMC7 in the diagnostic scoring system. However, our recent data have shown that CD20 is expressed, albeit weakly, in most CLL cases and that substitution of FMC7 by CD20 in the scoring system decreases significantly its diagnostic power (Delgado *et al.* 2003).

Prognostic impact of immunological markers

Beyond the diagnostic value of the membrane markers, immunophenotypic analysis has been shown to be useful for: (i) minimal residual disease detection; and (ii) estimating prognosis because the expression of certain molecules such as CD38, ZAP-70 and p53 seem to be associated with a poor outcome as described below.

CD38 expression has been shown in most studies to have a prognostic impact in CLL as a predictor for survival and disease progression. Although it was initially considered as a surrogate marker for IgVH mutational status (Damle *et al.* 1999), it has become apparent that it is an independent prognostic variable (Del Poeta *et al.* 2000; Ibrahim *et al.* 2001; Matrai *et al.* 2001). The technology used to detect CD38 in the cell membrane, the cut-off point to consider a case positive and the heterogeneity of patients included in the various studies may account for the discrepancies in the reported data. At present, it seems that a triple-colour flow cytometry to estimate the CD38 expression in B-cells from CLL and a cut-off point of 7% positive CLL cells is the optimal and more accurate (Figure 4.6).

ZAP-70 is a recently recognised marker with major prognostic implications in CLL. It is a member of a protein kinase family that has a variety of key functions, namely initiating T-cell signalling in T lymphocytes and in natural killer (NK) cells. This protein is strongly expressed in T and NK cells and weakly in B-cells. Gene expression profiling by microarray analysis first showed that ZAP-70 was differently expressed in CLL cases with unmutated IgVH compared to those with mutated IgVH (Klein *et al.* 2001; Rosenwald *et al.* 2001; Chen *et al.* 2002). This finding suggested that ZAP-70 could be a good discriminatory marker to distinguish between these two groups. More recently, a few studies using a McAb against ZAP-70 strongly suggest that ZAP-70 may well be a surrogate marker for Ig mutational status (Crespo *et al.* 2003). Nevertheless, there is still a need for standardisation to assess this marker and

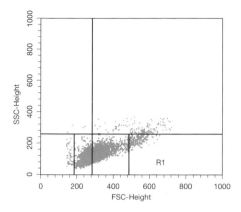

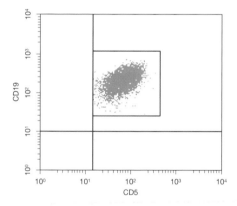

Gate: G1
X Parameter: CD5 (Log)
Y Parameter: CD19 (Log)

Quad	Events	% Gated	% Total
UL	0	0.00	0.00
UR	4332	100.00	86.64
LL	0	0.00	0.00
LR	0	0.00	0.00

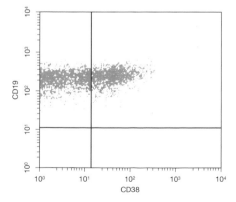

Gate: G1
X Parameter: CD38 (Log)
Y Parameter: CD19 (Log)

Quad	Events	% Gated	% Total
UL	2493	57.55	49.86
UR	1839	42.45	36.78
LL	0	0.00	0.00
LR	0	0.00	0.00

Figure 4.6 Dot plot from a case of CLL showing than greater than 50% of CLL cells (CD19⁺/CD5⁺) co-express CD38.

to establish clinically meaningful cut-off points to consider a result positive. From the technological point of view, ideally, ZAP-70 should be estimated by four-colour flow cytometry labelling using five McAb conjugated to different fluorochromes to discriminate objectively the T (CD3) and NK (CD56) cells from the B-CLL cells (CD5$^+$/CD19$^+$) that are ZAP-70 positive.

P53 abnormalities have been shown to have a major impact in clinical outcome in a variety of malignancies and, in CLL, to be associated with progressive disease, resistance to purine analogues and increase in prolymphocytes (CLL/PL) (Lens *et al.* 1997; Cordone *et al.* 1998; Dohner *et al.* 1995; Thornton *et al.* 2003). Abnormalities of p53 can be detected by several methods such as protein overexpression by flow cytometry, gene deletion by FISH or by gene sequencing to detect mutations. The latter, however, is a laborious technique which is not feasible on a routine basis. As it appears that there is a good correlation among the three methods (Thornton *et al.* 2004), flow cytometry to estimate protein over-expression or FISH to detect gene deletion are good alternatives to apply in a routine practice because of their simplicity and feasibility.

Diagnosis of difficult cases

Histology and/or FISH analysis are important tools in cases in which the diagnosis of CLL is uncertain due to the fact that cells are atypical morphologically or have an unusual immunophenotype.

Histology

Lymph node or tissue histology is only available in a few CLL cases because a substantial proportion of patients present with stage A disease without palpable nodes, and/or this investigation is not routinely performed unless Richter's transformation is suspected. In the latter situation, lymph node biopsy should always be performed.

In contrast, bone marrow histology can be easily available in all cases. Although the pattern of infiltration varies from diffuse, nodular or mixed (interstitial and nodular), there are some features that are helpful to differentiate CLL from other B-cell disorders. For instance, the presence of proliferating centres is a well recognised feature of CLL while is not seen in MCL; on the other hand, paratrabecular infiltration is exceptional in CLL but it is seen in a variety of B-cell lymphomas, in particular but not exclusively, follicular lymphoma. Further, immunohistochemistry using various McAb in particular, anti-cyclin D1 and bcl-6, may help further in the diagnosis.

Beyond the diagnostic value, bone marrow histology has a prognostic impact, with the diffuse pattern versus all the others correlating with poor outcome. The pure nodular pattern of bone marrow infiltration is rare in CLL, but it is seen more often today in patients treated with purine analogues or combinations who achieve a complete clinical response. In addition, bone marrow is useful to estimate or understand the mechanisms of cytopenias in CLL, for example whether due to hypersplenism or autoimmune phenomena or derived from progressive CLL and therefore it is recommended to be performed in all patients.

FISH/cytogenetics

Although these investigations are essentially performed for prognostic purposes, they are helpful in those cases in which the diagnosis of CLL is uncertain, e.g. atypical morphology and immunophenotype. Because low-grade lymphomas and particularly CLL have a low mitotic yield, FISH using probes that specifically detect certain chromosomal changes has replaced standard cytogenetics which is only performed in selected cases. From the practical point of view, FISH probes that allow us to distinguish CLL from certain B-cell lymphomas are those that detect t(11;14) (q13;q32) characteristic of MCL and t(14;18) typical of follicular lymphoma. Detection of trisomy 12 may help too, as it is frequently present in atypical CLL and CLL/PL. However, this abnormality on its own is not sufficient to establish the diagnosis of CLL, as it is seen as a secondary event in a proportion of MCL and other lymphomas. Likewise other abnormalities such as del13q14, del11q23 and del17p (p53), although seen in CLL, are not specific and are documented in other B-cell malignancies; thus, they lack diagnostic value despite of their relevant prognostic impact.

Differential diagnosis

The differential diagnosis of CLL arises with both primary leukaemias and B-cell lymphomas presenting with leukaemia, the latter likely underdiagnosed in the past.

CLL, and essentially CLL/PL, needs to be distinguished from B-PLL. Unlike CLL/PL in which there is a mixture of small and prolymphocytoid cells, in B-PLL the small-cell component is not seen and the main population corresponds to prolymphocytes with condensed but not clumped chromatin and a prominent single nucleolus. CLL scores in B-PLL are usually under 3.

When considering lymphomas, problems of differential diagnosis arise between CLL, both typical and atypical forms, and splenic lymphoma with villous lymphocytes (SLVL) or marginal zone lymphoma, lymphoplasmacytic lymphoma, MCL and follicular lymphoma. A final diagnosis is achieved in these cases when cell morphology and immunophenotype are compounded with FISH and/or histology.

Conclusions

CLL is a distinct chronic B-cell leukaemia. Clinical features together with examination of the lymphocyte morphology and immunophenotype are the two solid benchmarks that enable us to establish the diagnosis of CLL in most cases and rule out other B-cell disorders and reactive lymphocytosis. These investigations can easily be applied in the routine practice. The minority of cases with 'atypical' features may require further investigations, essentially cytogenetics/FISH and/or histology. Several of these tests not only provide relevant diagnostic information but also have been shown to have a prognostic impact. A precise diagnosis of CLL is important for the patient's management and to ascertain prognosis and disease outcome.

References

Alfarano, A., Indraccolo, S., Circosta, P. et al. (1999). An alternatively spliced form of CD79b gene may account for altered B-cell receptor expression in B-cell chronic lymphocytic leukemia. *Blood* **93**, 2327–2335.

Brito-Babapulle, V., Ellis, J., Matutes, E. et al. (1992) Translocation t(11;14)(q13;q32) in chronic lymphoid disorders. *Genes, Chromosomes and Cancer* **5**, 158–165.

Bennett, J. M., Catovsky, D., Daniel, M. T. et al. (1989). The French–American–British (FAB) Cooperative group. Proposals for the classification of chronic (mature) B and T lymphoid leukemias. *Journal of Clinical Pathology* **42**, 567–584.

Caligaris-Cappio, F. (1996) B-chronic lymphocytic leukemia: a malignancy of anti-self B cells. *Blood* **87**, 2615–2620.

Chen, L., Windhopf, G., Huynh, L. et al. (2002) Expression of ZAP-70 is associated with increased B-cell receptor signaling in chronic lymphocytic leukemia. *Blood* **100**, 4609–4614.

Cordone, I., Matutes, E. & Catovsky, D. (1992). Monoclonal antibody Ki-67 identifies B and T cells in cycle in chronic lymphocytic leukemia: correlation with disease activity. *Leukemia* **6**, 902–906.

Cordone, I., Masi, S., Mauro, F. R. et al. (1998). p53 expression in B-cell chronic lymphocytic leukemia: a marker of disease progression and poor prognosis. *Blood* **91**, 4342–4349.

Crespo, M., Bosch, F., Villamor, N. et al. (2003). ZAP-70 expression as a surrogate for Immunoglobulin variable region mutations in chronic lymphocytic leukemia. *New England Journal of Medicine* **348**, 1764–1775.

Criel, A., Wlodarska, I., Meeus, P. et al. (1994) Trisomy 12 is uncommon in typical chronic lymphocytic leukaemia. *British Journal of Haematology* **87**, 523–528.

Cuneo A., Balboni M., Piva N., et al. (1995). Atypical chronic lymphocytic leukaemia with t(11;14)(q13;q32): karyotype evolution and prolymphocytic transformation. *British Journal of Haematology* **90**, 409–416.

Cuneo A., Bigoni R., Negrini M. et al. (1997). Cytogenetic and interphase cytogenetic characterisation of atypical chronic lymphocytic leukemia carrying bcl-1 translocation. *Cancer Research* **57**, 1144–1150.

Damle, R. N., Wasil, T., Fais, F. et al. (1999). Immunoglobulin V gene mutation status and CD38 expression as novel prognostic indicators in chronic lymphocytic leukemia. *Blood* **94**, 1840–1847.

Delgado, J., Matutes, E., Morilla, A. M., Morilla, R. M., Owusu-Ankomah, K. A., Rafiq-Mohammed, F., del Giudice, I. & Catovsky, D. (2003) Diagnostic significance of CD20 and FMC7 expression in B-cell disorders. *American Journal of Clinical Pathology* **120**, 754–759.

Del Poeta, G., Maurillo, L., Venditti, A. et al. (2000) CD38 expression identifies two distinct prognostic subsets in B-chronic lymphocytic leukaemia. *Blood* **96** (Suppl. 1), 355a (abstract).

Dohner, H., Fischer, K., Bentz, M. et al. (1995). p53 gene deletion predicts poor survival and non-response to therapy with purine analogs in chronic B-cell leukemias. *Blood* **85**, 1580–1589.

Hamblin, T. J., Davis, Z., Gardiner, A. *et al.* (1999) Unmutated immunoglobulin VH genes are associated with a more aggressive form of chronic lymphocytic leukemia. *Blood* **94**, 1848–1854.

Ibrahim, S., Keating, M., Do, K.-A. *et al.* (2001) CD38 expression as an important prognostic factor in B-cell chronic lymphocytic leukemia. *Blood* **98**, 181–186.

Klein, U., Tu, Y., Stolovitzky, G. A. *et al.* (2001). Gene expression profiling of B cell chronic lymphocytic leukemia reveals a homogeneous phenotype related to memory cells. *Journal of Experimental Medicine* **194**, 1625–1638.

Lens, D., Dyer, M. J., Garcia-Marco, J. A. *et al.* (1997). p53 abnormalities in CLL are associated with excess of prolymphocytes and poor prognosis. *British Journal of Haematology* **99**, 848–857.

Matrai, Z., Lin, K., Dennis, M. *et al.* (2001) CD38 expression and IgVH gene mutation in B-cell chronic lymphocytic leukemia. *Blood* **97**, 1902–1903.

Matutes, E., Owusu-Ankomah, K., Morilla, R. *et al.* (1994). The immunological profile of B-cell disorders and proposal of a scoring system for the diagnosis of CLL. *Leukemia* **8**, 1640–1645.

Matutes, E. (1995). Contribution of immunophenotype in the diagnosis and classification of haemopoietic malignancies. *Journal of Clinical Pathology* **48**, 194–197.

Matutes, E., Oscier, D., Garcia Marco, J. *et al.* (1996) Trisomy 12 defines a group of CLL with atypical morphology. Correlation between cytogenetic, clinical and laboratory features in 544 patients. *British Journal of Haematology* **92**, 382–388.

Matutes, E., Halsey, J., Morilla, R. *et al.* (1999a) Prognostic significance of membrane antigens and morphology in chronic lymphocytic leukemia. *Blood* **94**, 535a (abstract).

Matutes, E., Carrara, P., Coignet, L. *et al.* (1999b). FISH analysis for BCL-1 rearrangements and trisomy 12 helps the diagnosis of atypical B cell leukaemias. *Leukemia* **13**, 1721–1726.

Matutes, E. & Polliack, A. (2000). Morphological and immunophenotypic features of chronic lymphocytic leukaemia. *Reviews of Clinical and Experimental Hematology* **4**, 22–47.

Matutes, E. (2002) New additions to antibody panels in the characterisation of chronic lymphoproliferative disorder. *Journal of Clinical Pathology* **55**, 180–183.

Michaux, L., Dierlamm, J., Wlodarska, I. *et al.* (1997) t(14;19)/BCL3 rearrangements in lymphoproliferative disorders: a review of 23 cases. *Cancer Genetics and Cytogenetics* **94**, 36–43.

Oscier, D., Matutes, E., Copplestone, A. *et al.* (1997). Atypical morphology: an adverse prognostic factor for disease progression in stage A CLL independent of trisomy 12. *British Journal of Haematology* **98**, 934–939.

Oscier, D., Fegan, C., Hillmen, P. *et al.* (2004). Guidelines on the diagnosis and management of chronic lymphocytic leukaemia. *British Journal of Haematology* **125**, 294–317.

Rosenwald, A., Alizadeh, A. A., Widhorpf, G., Simon, R. *et al.* (2001). Relation of gene expression phenotype to immunoglobulin mutation genotype in B cell chronic lymphocytic leukemia. *Journal of Experimental Medicine* **194**, 1639–1647.

Thompson, A. A., Talley J. A., Do, H. N. *et al.* (1997). Aberrations of the B cell receptor B29 (CD79b) gene in chronic lymphocytic leukemia. *Blood* **90**, 1387–1394.

Thornton, P. D., Gruszka-Westwood, A. M., Hamoudi, R. A., Atkinson, S., Kaczmarek, P., Morilla, R. M., Hilditch, B. L., A'Hern, R., Matutes, E. & Catovsky, D. (2004). Characterisation of TP53 abnormalities in chronic lymphocytic leukaemia. *Hematology Journal* **5**, 47–54.

Chapter 5

Modern prognostic factors: their impact on the treatment of early disease and the place of watchful waiting

Terry J. Hamblin

Introduction

For more than 25 years the CLL world has divided the disease into stages. The two classifications, Binet *et al.* (1977) and Rai *et al.* (1975), have been used consistently and chauvinistically depending on which side of the Atlantic Ocean one resides. For all intents and purposes they are interchangeable, and although there are minor differences, they have peacefully coexisted without the name-calling that the Atlantic Alliance has recently become familiar with. The details are given in Table 5.1. These classifications can be criticised. They should not be called stages, because that implies some sort of progression, and many cases do not progress. No direction is given on the causes of anaemia or thrombocytopenia, even though having a coincidental iron deficiency or even haemolytic anaemia does not carry the same grave prognosis as having advanced stage CLL. In addition it seems bizarre that the same levels of haemoglobin were chosen for men and women. A haemoglobin concentration of 11g/dl is much more severely reduced in a man than a woman.

Nevertheless, these systems have served the haematological community well for a long time and treatment decisions have been validly made by using them. Consistent survival differences between the different stages are seen (Table 5.1). A meta-analysis (CLL Trialists Collaborative Group 1991) has demonstrated that early treatment of early-stage disease produces no survival advantage over delaying treatment until progression occurs. However, the result of this meta-analysis depends on there being no better treatment for CLL than chlorambucil, and no way of knowing which early-stage cases are likely to progress. Neither of these suppositions is necessarily true. For example, the combination of fludarabine, cyclophosphamide and rituximab (Keating *et al.* 2003) produces much higher rates of complete remission in Phase II trials than does chlorambucil, and various prognostic systems purport to be able to pick winners from losers among early-stage patients.

A further important consideration is the fact that early-stage CLL is becoming commoner. Diagnostic guidelines have reduced the total lymphocyte count necessary to make the diagnosis, and making the diagnosis based on immunophenotype has further lowered the threshold. Recently, Rawstron *et al.* (2002a) suggested that 3.5%

of the population over the age of 40 had a monoclonal population of small lymphocytes immunophenotypically indistinguishable from CLL cells. The fact that such populations are much commoner among unaffected members of families in which familial CLL is established (Rawstron *et al.* 2002b) seems to confirm the truth of this observation.

Faced with an increasing number of patients with early-stage CLL, haematologists need better guidance on how they should be managed. Binet and Rai staging tell us about the bulk of disease present: what is needed is a means of distinguishing the biological nature of diseases.

Table 5.1 Rai and Binet staging

Rai	Characteristics	Survival
Stage 0	Lymphocytosis in blood and bone marrow only	12 years
Stage I	Lymphocytosis plus lymphadenopathy	7 years
Stage II	Lymphocytosis plus splenomegaly or hepatomegaly	
Stage III	Lymphocytosis plus anaemia, (Hb < 110 g/L)	
Stage IV	Lymphocytosis plus thrombocytopenia (platelets < 100×10^9/l)	< 1 year
*Binet**		
Stage A	< 3 sites involved, Hb > 100 g/l, platelets > 100 ¥ 10^9/l	9 years
Stage B	≥ 3 sites involved, Hb > 100 g/l, platelets > 100 ¥ 10^9/l	5 years
Stage C	Hb < 100 g/l, platelets > 100×10^9/l	2 years

*Involved sites are liver, spleen and lymph nodes in inguinal, axilliary and cervical regions.

Lymphocyte doubling time

The simplest means of determining whether or not CLL is progressing is to watch the white count. A lymphocyte doubling time of less than 12 months (Montserrat *et al.* 1986) is well correlated with progression, and indeed is used in the NCRI CLL4 trial as one of the means of recognising progressive stage A disease. However, there are caveats. Increases in lymphocyte counts are not necessarily linear. Especially if the patient is observed for only a short period and the doubling time calculated by extrapolation, errors may be unavoidable. Infection or immunisation or even exertion may temporarily raise the lymphocyte count and mislead. A further drawback is the need to watch for 12 months to be sure of the answer. In this time the patient may pass from curable to incurable.

Smouldering criteria

Workers in the field have long recognised that some patients with CLL have an indolent disease that seldom requires treatment. French and Spanish workers have sought to identify this cohort based on simple criteria available to all haematologists (French Cooperative Group on Chronic Lymphocytic Leukemia 1990; Montserrat *et al.* 1988). These criteria are given in Table 5.2. The Spanish called their cases smouldering CLL and the French Binet stage A'. These systems were designed to identify those patients who could safely be observed with little prospect of requiring treatment, but even the more stringent Spanish system misidentifies 25% of cases.

Table 5.2 Criteria for defining smouldering CLL

Spanish system
Binet stage A
Non-diffuse bone marrow histology
Hb > 13 g/dL
Lymphocyte count < 30×10^9/L
Lymphocyte doubling time > 12 months

French system
Binet stage A
Hb $\geq$ 12 g/dl
Lymphocyte count <30×10^9/l

Bone marrow histology

The Spanish group (Rozman *et al.* 1981) identified four patterns of involvement of bone marrow histology. Those patients with diffuse involvement of the bone marrow had a significantly worse prognosis than those with any other pattern. However, only one in six stage A patients have diffuse histology, and far more than this will require treatment. Furthermore, the histological pattern does not remain constant throughout the course of the disease, and serial bone marrow trephine biopsies are not received well by most patients.

Serum levels of soluble factors

Several soluble factors of prognostic import may be measured in the serum. Although they may to some degree be increased by disease proliferation, they also increased by increase in the tumour mass. Consequently, large volume, low activity disease may be indistinguishable from low volume, high activity disease. Those that are most popular in this context are CD23, thymidine kinase and β_2-microglobulin.

CD23

CD23 is the surface receptor for IgE and a useful diagnostic marker for CLL. It is rapidly cleaved from the cell surface to form a stable serum component. Although levels correlate with survival, the best correlations are obtained by following changes in level (Molica *et al.* 1996; Sarfati *et al.* 1996). This does not seem to offer much advantage over following changes in lymphocyte count, and no-one has adopted it as a useful indicator in the UK.

Thymidine kinase

Thymidine kinase is an enzyme involved in the preparation for cell division. Serum levels >7 U/L correlate well with progression in stage A CLL Hallek *et al.* 1999). However, only one in six patients have levels above 7 U/L. Levels are measured by radioimmunoassay. Radioactive isotopes are unwelcome in most UK laboratories.

β_2-microglobulin

β_2-microglobulin is a useful prognostic indicator in most types of lymphoma, and CLL is no exception. Thus far, it has been little used in the UK. In one study it added no prognostic information to CD38 expression (Ibrahim *et al.* 2001).

Karyotype

There are five common chromosomal abnormalities seen in CLL (Juliusson *et al.* 1990; Dohner *et al.* 2000). Deletion of part of the long arm of chromosome 13 (del 13q14) is the commonest, occurring in over 50% of cases. Patients with this deletion have a good prognosis, with survival curves that are even better than those with a normal karyotype. Trisomy 12 is the next commonest, occurring in up to 25% of cases. It is associated with atypical morphology and unmutated IgVH genes, and carries a worse than average prognosis. Deletions at 11q23 occur in about 10% of cases (Dohner *et al.* 1997,). Frequently the *ATM* (ataxia telangectasia mutated) gene is deleted. Because this gene is involved in the p53 pathway (Lin *et al.* 2002), its loss might be expected to have a malign effect. Cases are almost confined to the unmutated subset (see below) but such cases have a slightly worse prognosis than average for that subset. Deletions of 17p13 are only part of a larger group of patients with aberrations of the p53 gene detectable in a variety of ways (Dohner *et al.* 1995, Oscier *et al.* 2002; Krober *et al.* 2002). They occur in rather fewer than 10% of cases, depending on patient selection. Patients carrying p53 aberrations have the worst prognosis of all. Survival of less than 2 years is commonplace. Diverse deletions of part of the long arm of chromosome 6 occur in 6% of cases, but are usually secondary events.

Few laboratories are able to study karyotype efficiently, but the introduction of interphase fluorescent *in situ* hybridisation (FISH) has enabled this technique to become a vital part of the work-up of patients with CLL.

IgVH mutations

CLL was previously thought to be a tumour derived from naïve follicular mantle cells. Most cases had germ-line immunoglobulin genes (Kipps *et al.* 1989). The process of somatic hypermutation occurs within the germinal centre, and is used to improve the goodness-of-fit of antibody to antigen. Contact of a B lymphocyte with antigen in the context of T cells and antigen presenting cells in the germinal centre triggers a series of divisions in which mutating enzymes are active. Cells expressing antibody that fits well with the antigen are preserved and exit the germinal centre as memory B cells or proceed to the bone marrow to become plasma cells secreting the desired antibody. Cells expressing poorly-fitting antibody enter apoptosis.

A review by Schroeder and Dighiero (1994) found that 50% of reported CLLs had mutated IgVH genes, which was against the accepted dogma. Despite the fact that some of the reported cases proved not to be true cases of CLL, further studies proved that the observation was correct. Furthermore, two studies published simultaneously (Hamblin *et al.* 1999; Damle *et al.* 1999) demonstrated that patients with mutated IgVH genes had a median survival of about 25 years, while those with unmutated IgVH genes had a median survival of 8 years. These observations have been subsequently confirmed by other authors (Stilgenbauer 2002), and form the basis for a substantial division of the disease into two subtypes. Patients with mutated IgVH genes tend to have stable disease, typical morphology, stage A disease, and an equal distribution between the sexes. On the other hand those with unmutated IgVH genes tend to have progressive disease, atypical morphology, advanced stage disease and to be predominantly male (Hamblin *et al.* 2002).

The two subgroups differ in other ways. Although response to treatment seems to be similar in both subtypes (except for tumours with aberrations of the p53 pathway, which are usually resistant to both fludarabine and chlorambucil), in our series survival after the first treatment is twice as long in the mutated subset as in the unmutated subset. Following stem cell autograft, all cases with unmutated IgVH genes had relapsed molecularly by four years and most had relapsed clinically, whereas only a few had relapsed molecularly in the mutated subset and none clinically at four years (Ritgen *et al.* 2003). Although there is a general feeling that the disease is more malignant in younger patients, in our series the ratio of mutated to unmutated is the same for every decade of life. An important observation from our series is that the survival curve for stage A unmutated cases is parallel to that for stage B and C unmutated cases, but delayed for one year. In other words, any attempt to treat early before progression occurs cannot be long delayed.

There is a biased usage of the 51 possible VH genes (Chiorazzi & Ferrarini 2003). V1-69 is the most commonly used gene. Most cases are unmutated, and also use the D3-3 segment and the JH6 gene. Consequently, all such cases have similar antibody combining sites, and this implies the involvement of a specific antigen in the aetiology of CLL. This is also seen in cases using the V3-21 gene (Tobin *et al.* 2002, 2003). Here the D segment gene is nibbled away almost to nothing, and the same JH6 gene is used. Although the majority of cases are mutated, they still have strikingly similar antibody combining sites. Despite being mutated, the prognosis in this group is as poor as that of the unmutated subset. The third instance of nearly identical antibody combining sites concerns the unusual class-switched surface IgG positive CLLs (Chiorazzi & Ferrarini 2003). Some of these cases use the V4-39 gene and the D6-13 and JH5 gene segments. These cases are unmutated despite the fact that class switching and somatic mutations are both initiated by the same activation induced cytidine deaminase enzyme.

CD38

Despite its importance as a prognostic marker, detecting IgVH somatic mutations is too difficult an assay for routine use. A search for surrogate markers began when Damle *et al.* (1999) suggested that expression of surface CD38 detected by flow cytometry gives the same answers as IgVH mutations. Subsequent studies showed that there was a 30% discordance between CD38 positivity and unmutated IgVH genes (Hamblin *et al.* 2001; Stilgenbauer *et al.* 2002). This situation was further complicated by the discovery that CD38 expression can vary over time, principally because chemotherapy selectively kills CD38 negative cells, but also because there is a suggestion that intercurrent illness may be related to increases in CD38 expression on CLL cells (Hamblin *et al.* 2002). This increase may be related to in vivo secretion of γ-interferon or interleukin-2, both of which may induce CD38 expression in vitro (Deaglio *et al.* 2003).

A further interesting observation is that CD38 positivity predicts a shortened overall survival far better than it predicts early death from CLL, again pointing to the possibility that CD38 expression may be raised in patients with other life-threatening disease. Patients who are discordant for CD38 positivity and IgVH mutations have an intermediate median survival of about 15 years. Thus one paper (Hamblin *et al.* 2002) found that CD38 was an independent prognostic factor, but when this series was extended and karyotype added to the range of prognostic tests, this independence was lost (Oscier *et al.* 2002).

Microarrays

Two papers published in the same edition of the *Journal of Experimental Medicine* reported on the gene expression profile of CLL (Klein *et al.* 2001; Rosenwald *et al.* 2001). Both found that the genes expressed by both subsets were extremely similar, and very different from other types of lymphoma. However, a small group of genes (about 30 in 12,000) was expressed differently. Further investigations have increased this number to over 100 genes and one in particular, *ZAP-70*, is capable of segregating the two subtypes by itself. This gene codes for the zeta chain associated protein, part of the T-cell receptor complex, and therefore microarray investigations must be prefaced by depletion of T-cells and NK-cells from the test sample.

One of the papers investigated the possible cell of origin of CLL (Klein *et al.* 2001). The gene expression profile was more similar to non-germinal centre cells than to germinal centre cells. The attempt to allocate an origin to naïve or memory cells was not wholly successful, for 14 out of 20 samples the profile was significantly more like that of memory cells than naïve cells.

ZAP-70

Expression of *ZAP-70* is detectable by microarray or RT-PCR, and the protein may be detected by Western blotting or immunohistochemistry. None of these techniques is suitable for the routine laboratory, either requiring a T-cell depletion step or being only semi-quantitative (Wiestner *et al.* 2003). Flow cytometry has proved a more elusive assay to establish, but two groups have published assays (Crespo *et al.* 2003; Orchard *et al.* 2003). In both series concordance with IgVH gene mutations is about 90%, but those poor prognosis cases with mutated V3-21 genes seem to be ZAP-70 positive. Unfortunately as these series have expanded the concordance has become smaller, though cases with <95% IgVH homology are almost always ZAP-70 negative and cases with ≥ 99% homology are nearly always ZAP-70 positive. Cases with 95–98% homology are clearly an intermediate group, and this group warrants further study.

Conclusions

No single assay for prognosis is ideal. Estimation of IgVH gene mutations is the best, but it is cumbersome to perform. ZAP-70 expression is not yet fully evaluated. FISH gives additional information, especially about the likelihood of drug-resistant disease. All of the assays suffer from a lack of inter-laboratory quality control. Nevertheless, a combination of tests would usefully select patients for whom a prospective clinical trial would be an advantage.

Clinical Trials

Several groups have recognised the need for a new clinical trial in early-stage disease. The German and French groups have designed a randomised phase II study comparing early fludarabine, cyclophosphamide and rituximab with treatment delayed until progression in a group of high risk stage A patients. High risk is defined as a patient possessing two of the following: Unmutated IgVH genes, serum thymidine kinase level > 7 U/L, lymphocyte doubling time of less than 12 months or FISH indicating loss at 11q23 or 17p13.

The UK CLL forum has proposed phase II studies of two regimens in poor-risk early-stage CLL. Poor risk has been defined as having unmutated IgVH genes and CD38 expression of greater than 30%. In the first trial patients will receive 4 courses of oral fludarabine and cyclophosphamide. Patients in CR or nodular PR will pass to the next phase of treatment. Those not achieving this will receive two further courses, and those achieving PR or better will proceed to the second phase. This will consist of a three month wash-out period followed by 6 weeks of subcutaneous alemtuzumab 30 mg per week. The end points will be achievement of negative minimal residual disease as detectable by a four colour flow cytometric test and the detection of any adverse effects of the regimen. Using alemtuzumab after fludarabine has produced severe pancytopenia in a German pilot study, hence the need for the lowered dose and wash out period.

The second trial is in the same group of patients. This time the treatment will consist of six courses of fludarabine, cyclophosphamide and rituximab. The end points will be the same.

References

Binet, J.-L., Leporier, M., Dighiero, G., Carron, D., D'Athis, P. Vaugier, G., Merle Beral, H., Natali, J.C., Raphael, M., Nizit, N. G. & Follezlou, J. Y. (1977) A clinical staging system for chronic lymphocytic leukemia. *Cancer* **40**, 855–864.

Chiorazzi, N. & Ferrarini, M. (2003) B cell chronic lymphocytic leukemia: lessons learned from studies of the B cell antigen receptor. *Annual Reviews of Immunology* **21**, 841–894.

CLL Trialists Collaborative Group (1999). Chemotherapeutic options in chronic lymphocytic leukaemia: a meta-analysis of the randomised trials. *Journal of the National Cancer Institute* **91**, 861–868.

Crespo, M., Bosch, F., Villamor, N., Bellosillo, B., Colomer, D., Rozman, M., Marce, S., Lopez-Guillermo, A., Campo, E. & Montserrat, E. (2003). ZAP-70 expression as a surrogate for immunoglobulin-variable-region mutations in chronic lymphocytic leukemia. *New England Journal of Medicine* **348**, 1764–1775.

Damle, R. N., Wasil, T., Fais ,F., Ghiotto, F., Valetto, A., Allen, S.L., Buchbinder, A., Budman, D., Dittmar, K., Kolitz, J., Lichtman, S. M., Schulman, P., Vinciguerra, V. P., Rai, K. R., Ferrarini, M. & Chiorazzi, N. (1999). Ig V gene mutation status and CD38 expression as novel prognostic indicators in chronic lymphocytic leukemia. *Blood* **94**, 1840–1847.

Deaglio, S., Capobianco, A., Bergui, L., Durig, J., Morabito, F., Duhrsen, U. & Malavasi, F. (2003). CD38 is a signaling molecule in B-cell chronic lymphocytic leukemia cells. *Blood* **102**, 2146–2155.

Dohner, H., Stilgenbauer, S., Benner, A., Leupolt, E., Krober, A., Bullinger, L., Dohner, K., Bentz, M. & Lichter, P. (2000). Genomic aberrations and survival in chronic lymphocytic leukemia. *New England Journal of Medicine* **343**, 1910–1916.

Dohner, H., Stilgenbauer, S., James, M., Benner, A., Weilguni, T., Bentz, M., Fischer, K., Hunstein, W. & Lichter, P. I. (1997). 11q deletions identify a new subset of B-cell chronic lymphocytic leukemia characterised by extensive nodal involvement and inferior prognosis. *Blood* **89**, 2516–2522.

Dohner, H., Fischer, K., Bentz, M., Hansen, K., Benner, A., Cabot, G., Diehl, D., Schlenk, R., Coy, J., Stilgenbauer, S. & Lichter, P. I. (1995). p53 gene deletion predicts for poor survival and non-response to therapy with purine analogs in chronic B-cell leukemias. *Blood* **85**, 1580–1589.

French Cooperative Group on Chronic Lymphocytic Leukemia (1990). Natural history of stage A chronic lymphocytic leukemia untreated patients. *British Journal of Haematology* **76**, 45–57.

Hallek, M., Langenmayer, I., Neri, C., Knauf, W., Dietzfelbinger, H., Adorf, D., Ostwald, M., Busch, R., Kuhn-Hallek, I., Thiel, E. & Emmerich, B. (1999). Elevated serum thymidine kinase levels identify a subgroup at high risk of disease progression in early, nonsmouldering chronic lymphocytic leukemia. *Blood* **93**, 1732–1737

Hamblin, T. J., Davis, Z., Gardiner, A., Oscier, D. G. & Stevenson, F. K. (1999). Unmutated Ig V(H) genes are associated with a more aggressive form of chronic lymphocytic leukemia. *Blood* **94**, 1848–1854.

Hamblin, T. J., Orchard, J. A., Ibbotson, R. E., Davies, Z., Thomas, P. W., Stevenson, F. K. & Oscier, D. G. (2002). CD38 expression and immunoglobulin variable region mutations are independent prognostic variables in chronic lymphocytic leukemia, but CD38 expression may vary during the course of the disease. *Blood* **99**, 1023–1029.

Ibrahim, S., Keating, M., Do, K. A. Rogers, A., Manshouri, T., Giles, F., Faderl, S., Thomas, D., Kantarjian, H., Keating, M. & Albitar, M. (2001). CD38 expression as an important prognostic factor in B-cell chronic lymphocytic leukemia. *Blood* **98**, 181–186.

Juliusson, G., Oscier, D. G., Fitchett, M., Ross, F. M., Stockdill, G., Mackie, M. J., Parker, A. C., Castoldi, G. L., Guneo, A. & Knuutila, S. (1990). Prognostic subgroups in B-cell chronic lymphocytic leukemia defined by specific chromosomal abnormalities. *New England Journal of Medicine* **323**, 720–724

Keating, M. J., Chiorazzi, N., Messmer, B., Damle, R. N., Allen, S. L., Rai, K. R., Ferrarini, M. & Kipps, T. J. (2003). Biology and treatment of chronic lymphocytic leukemia. *Hematology (American Society of Hematology Education Program)*, 153–175.

Kipps, T. J., Tomhave, E., Pratt, L. F., Duffey, S., Chen, P. P. & Carson, D. A. (1989). Developmentally restricted immunoglobulin heavy chain variable region gene expressed at high frequency in chronic lymphocytic leukemia. *Proceedings of the National Academy of Science of the United States of America* **86**, 5913–5917.

Klein, U., Tu, Y., Stolovitzky, G. A., Mattioli, M., Cattoretti, G., Husson, H., Freedman, A., Inghirami, G., Cro, L., Baldini, L., Neri, A., Califano, A. & Dalla-Favera, R. (2001). Gene expression profiling of B cell chronic lymphocytic leukemia reveals a homogeneous phenotype related to memory B cells. *Journal of Experimental Medicine* **194**, 1625–1638.

Krober, A., Seller, T., Benner, A., Bullinger, L., Bruckle, E., Lichter, P., Dohner, H. & Stilgenbauer, S. (2002). V_H mutation status, CD38 expression level, genomic aberrations, and survival in chronic lymphocytic leukemia. *Blood* **100**, 1410–1416.

Lin, K., Sherrington, P. D., Dennis, M., Matrai, Z., Cawley, J.C. & Pettitt, A. R. (2002). Relationship between p53 dysfunction, CD38 expression, and IgV(H) mutation in chronic lymphocytic leukemia. *Blood* **100**, 1404–1409.

Molica, S., Levato, D., Dell'Olio, M., Matera, R., Minervini, M., Dattilo, A., Carotenuto, M. & Musto, P. (1996). Cellular expression and serum circulating levels of CD23 in B-cell chronic lymphocytic leukemia. Implications for prognosis. *Haematologica* **81**, 428–433.

Montserrat, E., Sanchez-Bisono, J., Vinolas, N. & Rozman, C. (1986). Lymphocyte doubling time in chronic lymphocytic leukaemia: analysis of its prognostic significance. *British Journal of Hematology* **62**, 567–575.

Montserrat, E., Vinolas, N., Reverter, J. C. & Rozman, C. (1988). Natural history of chronic lymphocytic leukemia: on the progression and prognosis of early stages. *Nouvelle Revue Francais Hematologie* **30**, 359–361.

Orchard, J. A., Ibbotson, R. E., Davis, Z., Wiestner, A., Rosenwald, R., Thomas, P. W., Hamblin, T. J., Staudt, L. M. & Oscier, D. G. (2004). ZAP-70 expression by flow cytometry is a good prognostic marker in CLL and a potential surrogate for immunoglobulin *VH* gene mutations. *The Lancet* **363**, 105–111.

Oscier, D. G., Gardiner, A. C., Mould, S. J., Glide, S., Davies, Z. A., Ibbotson, R. E., Corcoran, M. M., Chapman, R. M., Thomas, P. W., Copplestone, J. A., Orchard, J. A. & Hamblin T. J. (2002). Multivariate analysis of prognostic factors in CLL: Clinical stage, *IGVH* gene mutational status, and loss or mutation of the *p53* gene are independent prognostic factors. *Blood* **100**, 1177–1184.

Rai, K. R., Sawitsky, A., Cronkite, E. R., Chanana, A. D., Levy, R. N. & Pasternack, B. S. (1975). Clinical staging of chronic lymphocytic leukemia. *Blood* **46**, 219–234.

Rawstron, A. C., Green, M. J., Kuzmicki, A., Kennedy, B., Fenton, J. A., Evans, P. A., O'Connor, S. J., Richards, S. J., Morgan, G. J., Jack, A. S. & Hillmen P. (2002a). Monoclonal B lymphocytes with the characteristics of "indolent" chronic lymphocytic leukemia are present in 3.5% of adults with normal blood counts. *Blood.* **100**, 635–639.

Rawstron, A. C., Yuille, M. R., Fuller, J., Cullen, M., Kennedy, B., Richards, S. J., Jack, A. S., Matutes, E., Catovsky, D., Hillmen, P. & Houlston, R. S. (2002b). Inherited predisposition to CLL is detectable as subclinical monoclonal B-lymphocyte expansion. *Blood* **100**, 2289–2290.

Ritgen, M., Lange, A., Stilgenbauer, S., Dohner, H., Bretscher, C., Bosse, H., Stuhr, A., Kneba, M. & Dreger, P. (2003). Unmutated immunoglobulin variable heavy-chain gene status remains an adverse prognostic factor after autologous stem cell transplantation for chronic lymphocytic leukemia. *Blood* **101**, 2049–2053.

Rosenwald, A., Alizadeh, A. A., Widhopf, G., Simon, R., Davis, R. E., Yu, X., Yang, L., Pickeral, O. K., Rassenti, L. Z., Powell, J., Botstein, D., Byrd, J. C., Grever, M. R., Cheson, B. D., Chiorazzi, N., Wilson, W. H., Kipps, T. J., Brown, P. O. & Staudt, L. M. (2001). Relation of gene expression phenotype to immunoglobulin mutation genotype in B cell chronic lymphocytic leukemia. *Journal of Experimental Medicine* **194**, 1639–1647.

Rozman, C., Hernandez-Nieto, L., Montserrat, E. & Brugues, R. (1981). Prognostic significance of bone marrow patterns in chronic lymphocytic leukaemia. *British Journal of Haematology* **47**, 529-537

Sarfati, M., Chevet, S. Chastang, C., Biron, G., Stryckmans, P., Delespesse, G., Binet, J. L., Merle-Beral, H. & Bron, D. (1996). Prognostic importance of serum levels of CD23 in chronic lymphocytic leukemia. *Blood* **88**, 4259–4264.

Schroeder, H.W. Jr & Dighiero, G. (1994). The pathogenesis of chronic lymphocytic leukemia: analysis of the antibody repertoire. *Immunology Today* **15**, 288–294.

Stilgenbauer, S., Bullinger, L., Lichter, P. & Dohner, H.; German CLL Study Group (GCLLSG) (2002). Chronic lymphocytic leukemia. Genetics of chronic lymphocytic leukemia: genomic aberrations and V(H) gene mutation status in pathogenesis and clinical course. *Leukemia* **16**, 993–1007.

Tobin, G., Thunberg, U., Johnson, A., Thorn, I., Soderberg, O., Hultdin, M., Botling, J., Enblad, G., Sallstrom, J., Sundstrom, C., Roos, G. & Rosenquist, R. (2002). Somatically mutated IgV$_H$3-21 genes characterize a new subset of chronic lymphocytic leukemia. *Blood* **99**, 2262–2264.

Tobin, G., Thunberg, U., Johnson, A., Eriksson, I., Soderberg, O., Karlsson, K., Merup, M., Juliusson, G., Vilpo, J., Enblad, G., Sundstrom, C., Roos, G. & Rosenquist. R. (2003). Chronic lymphocytic leukemias utilizing the VH3-21 gene display highly restricted V lambda 2-14 gene use and homologous CDR3s: implicating recognition of a common antigen epitope. *Blood* **101**, 4952–4957.

Wiestner, A., Rosenwald, A., Barry, T. S., Wright, G., Davis, R. E., Henrickson, S. E., Zhao, H., Ibbotson, R. E., Orchard, J. ., Davis, Z., Stetler-Stevenson, M., Raffeld, M., Arthur, D. C., Marti, G. E., Wilson, W. H., Hamblin, T. J., Oscier, D. G. & Staudt, L. M. (2003). ZAP-70 expression identifies a chronic lymphocytic leukemia subtype with unmutated immunoglobulin genes, inferior clinical outcome, and distinct gene expression profile. *Blood* **101**, 4944–4951.

Chapter 6

First line medical intervention in chronic lymphocytic leukaemia

Bruno Cazin

Introduction

Despite a life expectancy of longer than 10 years in early-stage patients, patients with advanced B-cell chronic lymphocytic leukaemia (B-CLL) have a shorter median survival, typically between 18 months and 3 years (Binet *et al.* 1981, Rai *et al.* 1975). Apart from classical clinical prognostic factors, both the IgV mutation status and the pattern of genomic aberrations led to an improved knowledge of prognostic factors in B-CLL. Therefore, therapeutic approaches are currently being reassessed, especially the benefit of an early treatment for patients with poor prognostic factors. The rule of maintaining a watch-and-wait policy in the early stage disease of CLL is now open to debate. It was based on clinical data of large studies (Dighiero *et al.* 1998) and confirmed by a meta-analysis (CLL Group 1999) on therapies based on alkylating agents, which rarely result in complete remissions. In this chapter, I consider that the choice to initiate treatment in the patient with B-CLL, from clinical trials, is based on clinical evidence for active disease (Cheson *et al.* 1996), and from new prognostic factors (cytogenetics, mutational status of IgVH gene, biological parameters) whose impact is still being evaluated.

A wider therapeutic choice offers new approaches to the treatment of CLL. A high remission rate in first-line therapy is associated with longer progression-free survival, so that the choice of this treatment appears of greater importance. Eradication of minimal residual disease may be the optimal endpoint for younger patients. Whether these high-quality remissions translate into a significant survival advantage is still being investigated, though it is probable.

Alkylating agents

Alkylating agents alone or in combination were the standard treatments during recent decades. Chlorambucil is effective at palliating most CLL patients, but its benefit relative to overall survival compared with watch-and-wait is not established. Different schedules and dose-intensities of chlorambucil have been used (Table 6.1). Efficacy seems to be dose dependent.

Chlorambucil is frequently associated with prednisone, but the advantage of this association has not been demonstrated. Corticosteroids may increase the risk of infections in immunocompromised patients. Single-agent steroids may increase

Table 6.1 Current dosage and schedules of CLL treatments

Treatment	Way of administration	Dosage	Schedule	Reference
chlorambucil	oral	0.1 mg/kg daily 0.3 mg/kg d1–d5 monthly 15 mg total dose daily	until best response until toxicity or complete remission	Dighiero 1998 Jaksic & Brugiatelli 1988
miniCHOP	i.v. IV oral oral	Vincristine 1 mg/m^2 d1 maximum 2 mg Doxorubicin 25 mg/m^2 d1 Cyclophosphamide 300 mg/m^2/d d1–d5 Prednisone 40 mg/m^2/d d1–d5	every 28 days for 6 cycles	Leporrier et al. 2001
CAP	i.v. i.v. oral	Cyclophosphamide 750 mg/m^2/d1 Doxorubicin 50mg/m^2/d1 Prednisone 40 mg/m^2/d d1–d5	every 28 days for 6 cycles	CLL Group 1999; Johnson et al. 1996
fludarabine	i.v.	25 mg/m^2/d d1–d5	every 28 days for 6 cycles or best response	
fludarabine	oral	40 mg/m^2/d d1–d5	every 28 days for 6 cycles or best response	
fludarabine cyclophosphamide	i.v. i.v.	25 to 30 mg/m^2/d d1–d3 250 to 300 mg/m^2/d d1–d3	every 28 days for 6 cycles or best response	O'Brien et al. 2001b
fludarabine cyclophosphamide	oral oral	25 to 30 mg/m^2/d d1–d5 150 to 200 mg/m2/d d1–d5	every 28 days for 6 cycles or best response	Cazin et al. 2002
fludarabine cyclophosphamide mitoxantrone	i.v. i.v. i.v.	25 to 30 mg/m^2/d d1–d3 200 mg/m^2/d d1–d3 6 mg/m^2 i.v. d1	every 28 days for 6 cycles or best response	Bosch et al. 2002

hyperlymphocytosis and should not be proposed outside of the treatment of autoimmune complications of CLL.

Combination therapies including alkylating agents, corticosteroids and anthracycline (CAP, chlorambucil + epirubicin), alkylating agents, anthracyclines, vincristine and steroids (miniCHOP), alkylating agents, vincristine and steroids (COP) are used in CLL, but comparisons with chlorambucil regimens have never demonstrated superiority for prolonged survival.

Purine analogues

The advent of the purine analogues in the early 1990s, in particular of fludarabine phosphate, has had a major impact on the management of CLL. These agents include the adenosine deaminase inhibitors pentostatin, cladribine and fludarabine. Fludarabine has been the most extensively studied agent in CLL.

In first-line treatment, fludarabine allows a higher response rate and a longer progression-free survival compared with CAP (Johnson *et al.* 1996) or with chlorambucil (Rai *et al.* 2000) (Table 6.2). Fludarabine is quite possibly the most active single agent in CLL. The usual dose and schedule is 25mg/m^2/day by intravenous injection for five consecutive days every four weeks during six cycles. It achieved overall response rates (ORRs) of 63–71% and 8–23% complete remission (CR). However, the high response rate had no impact on survival in randomised comparative studies between fludarabine and chlorambucil or a polychemotherapy regimen, mainly because treatment cross-over is frequent (Leporrier *et al.* 2001) (Table 6.2). Myelosuppression and infections are slightly increased with fludarabine compared with an alkylating-based regimen, but alopecia was not observed.

Quality of life is improved with fludarabine (Levy *et al.* 2001) and life expectancy of advanced CLL is longer since the introduction of purine analogues compared with historical series. When the Binet stage was defined, based on the French CLL trial in 1976, median survival for stage B was 62 months and 24 months in stage C. In the CLL 90 trial published by Leporrier *et al.* (2001), median survival of stage B was 79 months, and 58.5 months in stage C. Studies on long-term follow up of patients treated with fludarabine indicate a slightly longer overall survival (Keating *et al.* 1998).

The results of these studies provide justification for using fludarabine as first-line therapy, which has been recently approved in Europe.

An oral formulation of fludarabine has been developed. Its efficacy does not differ from its intravenous formulation and its safety profile is quite similar (Boogaerts *et al.* 2001; Rossi *et al.* 2004). A dose of 40 mg/m^2 is equivalent to 25 mg/m^2 intravenously, and the 24 hour area under the concentration–time curve is similar for both formulations. Bioavailability is unaffected by food (Oscier *et al.* 2001).

Table 6.2 Phase III studies in CLL comparing fludarabine with conventional therapy

Study	Treatment	Patients	Overall response rate	Complete response rate	Mean PFS (months)	Mean OS (months)
(Rai et al. 1975)	Fludarabine (F) versus chlorambucil (C)	506 untreated	F: 63.0% C: 37.0% p < 0.001	F: 20% C: 3%	20 14	66 56
Johnson et al. 1996	F versus CAP	100 untreated	F: 71% CAP: 60% p: 0.026	F: 23% CAP: 17%	NR 7	NR 54
Leporrier et al. 2001	F versus CAP Versus CHOP	938 untreated	F: 71.1% CHOP: 71.5% CAP: 58.2% p < 0.001	F: 8% CHOP: 9% CAP: 2%	32 28 30	69 70 67

Fludarabine inhibits repair of DNA damage caused by agents such as mitoxantrone and cyclophosphamide (Kohl *et al.* 1997; Plunkett *et al.* 1993). A synergistic effect has been demonstrated *in vitro* and confirmed *in vivo* with the fludarabine–cyclophosphamide (FC) combination (Flinn *et al.* 2000; O'Brien *et al.* 2001b) (Table 6.3) and the triple combination of fludarabine, cyclophosphamide, mitoxantrone (FCM) (Bosch *et al.* 2002). Response rate and progression-free survival with combination therapy are higher than fludarabine alone, but no randomized trial has been yet published. Oral combination therapy of cyclophosphamide and fludarabine in a 5 day regimen every 28 days for 6 cycles in non-treated CLL patients demonstrated high response rate (80% ORR, 53.3% CR) (Cazin *et al.* 2003). Median DFS and survival are around 3 years. The combination of fludarabine with chlorambucil induced an important degree of myelosuppression and led to discontinuation in a large US trial (Rai *et al.* 2000).

Table 6.3 Fludarabine/cyclophosphamide regimens in untreated patients with CLL

Study	Number of patients	Regimen	ORR (%)	CR (%)
O'Brien *et al.* 2001b	34	F: 30mg/m^2 days 1–3 C: 300–500 mg/m^2 days 1–3	88	35
Flinn *et al.* 2000	36	F: 20 mg/m^2 days 1–5 C: 600 mg/m^2 day 1 plus G-CSF 5µg/kg days 8–18/22	64	42
Hallek *et al.* 2001	14	F: 30mg/m^2 days 1–3 C: 250 mg/m^2 days 1–3	83	21
Cazin *et al.* 2003	76	F: 30 mg/m^2 p.o. days 1–5 C: 200 mg/m^2 p.o. days 1–5	80	53
Keating *et al.* 2002	135	F: 25 mg/m^2 d1–3 C: 250 mg/m^2 d1–3 Rituximab 375–500 mg/m^2 d1	95	67

These good results of fludarabine combination therapy lead us to recommend its use in first-line therapy in younger patients, before the confirmation by phase III randomised trials for German (Eichhorst *et al.* 2003) and US groups.

The use of other purine analogues in the treatment of CLL has been more limited. Cladribine (Robak 2001) gives similar results to fludarabine. Cladribine and prednisone give a better CR rate, ORR and progression-free survival compared with chlorambucil and prednisone (Robak *et al.* 2000). The cladribine-cyclophosphamide (Robak *et al.* 2002) combination was tested in 82 previously untreated patients with advanced or progressive B-CLL, who received 2-CDA (cladribine) at a dose of 0.12 mg/kg for three consecutive days and CY at a dose of 650mg/m^2 on day 1 repeated every 4 weeks until maximum response. Overall response was 87.8% of whom 29.3%

had CR. Pentostatin as a single agent had less activity in a small phase II CALGB trial (Dillman *et al.* 1989). The combination of pentostatin and cyclophosphamide has only been tested in previously treated CLL (Weiss *et al.* 2003).

Despite high remission rates and long disease-free survival, chemotherapy alone cannot cure CLL. Almost all patients have detectable minimal residual disease (MRD) after the end of therapy and virtually all will experience a relapse. Complementary treatments targeted at eradicating MRD may lead to improved outcomes. Several studies focus on adding monoclonal antibodies to fludarabine-containing regimens.

Monoclonal antibodies

There are currently two monoclonal antibodies available for the treatment of B-cell malignancies: antiCD20 antibody (rituximab) and antiCD52 antibody (Campath-1H).

Alemtuzumab (Campath-1H) has been evaluated in previously untreated CLL patients (Lundin *et al.* 2002) with an overall response rate of 87% in 38 evaluable patients, including 18% CR. Alemtuzumab 30 mg was administered by subcutaneous injection thrice weekly for up to 18 weeks. This way of administration was well tolerated, with none of the infusion-related symptoms, only some local reactions at the site of injection. Fewer complications were observed in these chemotherapy-naive patients. Prolonged treatment (up to 18 weeks) was needed to obtain maximal response in bone marrow, lymph nodes and spleen. Alemtuzumab is relatively more active in blood, spleen and bone marrow than in lymph nodes, especially if they are bulky. Alemtuzumab is not indicated for first-line therapy of CLL, outside of clinical trials, but it is being studied for its ability to eliminate minimal residual disease after standard chemotherapy. Apart from immediate side effects related to cytokine release syndrome, alemtuzumab causes limited myelosuppression, principally neutropenia and prolonged immunosuppression with an important risk for cytomegalovirus reactivation and opportunistic infections. The use of alemtuzumab in monotherapy seems to be limited. It should be used as consolidation treatment after initial chemotherapy or in combination with chemotherapy. Various clinical studies are ongoing to determine its clinical benefit and the more appropriate dosage and schedule (Rai *et al.* 2002).

Rituximab alone showed some activity in the therapy of relapsed CLL, but its activity is dose dependent (Byrd *et al.* 2001; O'Brien *et al.* 2001a). There are still no data in the literature on rituximab as a single agent in symptomatic previously untreated CLL. However, rituximab administered concurrently with fludarabine in previously untreated patients demonstrates a better efficacy compared with sequential use (Byrd *et al.* 2003). In 20 previously untreated patients, 17 (85%) responded of whom 5 achieved CR (Schulz *et al.* 2002). The combination of fludarabine, cyclophosphamide and rituximab (FCR) leads to a high response rate (95% ORR and 67% CR in 135 patients) and molecular response (Keating *et al.* 2002).

Various combinations of monoclonal antibodies and antibodies with chemotherapy are being studied. Other monoclonal antibodies (antiHLA-DR, antiCD22 and antiCD23) are available for clinical studies in lymphoid malignancies.

However, a combination of chemotherapy with monoclonal antibodies, although improving response rates and disease-free survival, does not appear curative. Randomised trials are required to consider these combination therapies as standard treatment in younger patients.

Intensification as consolidation therapy

The possibilities offered by intensification with high-dose chemotherapy or radiotherapy with autologous stem-cell support and above all (non-myeloablative) allogeneic stem-cell transplantation allow us to shift the focus from palliation to cure. However, there is no plateau in the survival curves after autograft, despite prolonged MRD-negative observation. The benefit of early autologous stem-cell transplantation versus delayed transplantation is currently on study by the French Cooperative Group for CLL and should not be recommended before the result of this randomized trial is known. Except in very bad prognostic CLL in younger patients (who are refractory to treatment), allogeneic stem-cell transplantation should not be proposed in first-line treatment. Results and indications for intensification and transplantation are considered later in this volume.

Elderly patients

Newer therapeutic approaches to the management of CLL with the possibility of prolonged remission and cure in this disease, currently considered as uncurable, are very exciting. However, we should not forget that median age of diagnosis in CLL is 63 years and many patients are over 70. In elderly patients, the choice of first-line therapy may imbalance the clinical benefit and the potential toxicity, so that classical therapies with alkylating agents or fludarabine alone are still indicated. Palliation is still the goal of therapy in most patients, and the aim of the therapeutic choice will be to limit myelotoxicity and immune suppression to reduce infectious complications.

Conclusion

In conclusion, the choice of first-line medical intervention in CLL remains difficult. The spectrum is very broad, from chlorambucil to intensification with allogeneic stem-cell transplant, through purine analogues, monoclonal antibodies, to autologous stem-cell transplantation. In all patients, it is important to have a clear intent in choosing the first-line therapy for CLL: palliative (choice of the less toxic treatment) or curative (first choice of the best available combination or inclusion in clinical trials). Age, new prognostic factors, existence of a familial human leukocyte antigen (HLA) identical sibling, and the personal choice of the patient have to be taken into consideration.

References

Binet, J. L., Auquier, A., Dighiero, G., Chastang, C., Piguet, H., Goasguen, J., Vaugier, G., Potron, G., Colona, P., Oberling, F., Thomas, M., Tchernia, G., Jacquillat, C., Boivin, P., Lesty, C., Duault, M. T., Monconduit, M., Belabbes, S. & Gremy, F. (1981). A new prognostic classification of chronic lymphocytic leukemia derived from a multivariate survival analysis. *Cancer* **48**, 198–206.

Boogaerts, M. A., Van Hoof, A., Catovsky, D., Kovacs, M., Montillo, M., Zinzani, P. L., Binet, J. L., Feremans, W., Marcus, R., Bosch, F., Verhoef, G. & Klein, M. (2001). Activity of oral fludarabine phosphate in previously treated chronic lymphocytic leukemia. *Journal of Clinical Oncology* **19**, 4252–4258.

Bosch, F., Ferrer, A., Lopez-Guillermo, A., Gine, E., Bellosillo, B., Villamor, N., Colomer, D., Cobo, F., Perales, M., Esteve, J., Altes, A., Besalduch, J., Ribera, J. M. & Montserrat, E. (2002). Fludarabine, cyclophosphamide and mitoxantrone in the treatment of resistant or relapsed chronic lymphocytic leukaemia. *Brtish Journal of Haematology* **119**, 976–984.

Byrd, J. C., Murphy, T., Howard, R. S., Lucas, M. S., Goodrich, A., Park, K., Pearson, M., Waselenko, J. K., Ling, G., Grever, M. R., Grillo-Lopez, A. J., Rosenberg, J., Kunkel, L. & Flinn, I. W. (2001). Rituximab using a thrice weekly dosing schedule in B-cell chronic lymphocytic leukemia and small lymphocytic lymphoma demonstrates clinical activity and acceptable toxicity. *Journal of Clinical Oncology* **19**, 2153–2164.

Byrd, J. C., Peterson, B. L., Morrison, V. A., Park, K., Jacobson, R., Hoke, E., Vardiman, J. W., Rai, K., Schiffer, C. A. & Larson, R. A. (2003). Randomized phase 2 study of fludarabine with concurrent versus sequential treatment with rituximab in symptomatic, untreated patients with B-cell chronic lymphocytic leukemia: results from Cancer and Leukemia Group B 9712 (CALGB 9712). *Blood* **101**, 6–14.

Cazin, B. *et al.* (2002). Oral fludarabine and cyclophosphamide in previously untreated CLL: preliminary data on 75 patients (abstract). *Blood* **100**, 206a.

Cazin, B., Maloum, K., Divine, M., Leprêtre, S., Travade, P., Delmer, A., Jaubert, J., Lederlin, P., Dreyfus, B., Leporrier, M., Harousseau, M., Grosbois, B., Maloisel, F., Eghbali, H., Dumontet, C., Benichou, J. & Guibon, O. (2003). Oral fludarabine phosphate and cyclophosphamide in previously untreated CLL: final rsponse and follow up in 75 patients. *Blood* **102**(11), 438a (abstract).

Cheson, B. D., Bennett, J. M., Grever, M., Kay, N., Keating, M. J., O'Brien, S. & Rai, K. R. (1996). National Cancer Institute-sponsored Working Group guidelines for chronic lymphocytic leukemia: revised guidelines for diagnosis and treatment. *Blood* **87**, 4990–4997.

CLL Group (1999). Chemotherapeutic options in chronic lymphocytic leukemia: a meta-analysis of the randomized trials. CLL Trialists' Collaborative Group. *Journal of the National Cancer Institute* **91**, 861–868.

Dighiero, G., Maloum, K., Desablens, B., Cazin, B., Navarro, M., Leblay, R., Leporrier, M., Jaubert, J., Lepeu, G., Dreyfus, B., Binet, J. L. & Travade, P. (1998). Chlorambucil in indolent chronic lymphocytic leukemia. French Cooperative Group on Chronic Lymphocytic Leukemia. *New England Journal of Medicine* **338**, 1506–1514.

Dillman, R. O., Mick, R. & McIntyre, O. R. (1989). Pentostatin in chronic lymphocytic leukemia: a phase II trial of Cancer and Leukemia group B. *Journal of Clinical Oncology* **7**, 433–438.

Eichhorst, B., Busch, R., Hpfinger, G., Pasold, R., Hensel, M., Söling, U., Siehl, S., Steinbrecher, C., Jäger, U., Bergmann, M., Wendtner, C., Hiddemann, W., Emmerich, B. & Hallek, M. (2003). Fludarabine plus cyclophosphamide induces higher response rates and longer progression free survival (PFS) than fludarabine alone in first line therapy of advanced chronic lymphocytic leukemia (CLL): results of a phase II study (CLL4 protocol) of the German CLL study group (GCLLSG). *Blood* **102**(11), 72a (abstract).

Flinn, I. W., Byrd, J. C., Morrison, C., Jamison, J., Diehl, L. F., Murphy, T., Piantadosi, S., Seifter, E., Ambinder, R. F., Vogelsang, G. & Grever, M. R. (2000). Fludarabine and cyclophosphamide with filgrastim support in patients with previously untreated indolent lymphoid malignancies. *Blood* **96**, 71–75.

Hallek, M., Schmitt, B., Wilhelm, M., Busch, R., Krober, A., Fostitsch, H. P., Sezer, O., Herold, M., Knauf, W., Wendtner, C. M., Kuse, R., Freund, M., Franke, A., Schriever, F., Nerl, C., Dohner, H., Thiel, E., Hiddemann, W., Brittinger, G. & Emmerich, B. (2001). Fludarabine plus cyclophosphamide is an efficient treatment for advanced chronic lymphocytic leukaemia (CLL): results of a phase II study of the German CLL Study Group. *Brtish Journal of Haematology* **114**, 342–348.

Jaksic, B. & Brugiatelli, M. (1988). High dose continuous chlorambucil vs intermittent chlorambucil plus prednisone for treatment of B-CLL—IGCI CLL-01 trial. *Nouv Rev Fr Hematol,* **30**, 437–442.

Johnson, S., Smith, A. G., Loffler, H., Osby, E., Juliusson, G., Emmerich, B., Wyld, P. J. & Hiddemann, W. (1996). Multicentre prospective randomised trial of fludarabine versus cyclophosphamide, doxorubicin, and prednisone (CAP) for treatment of advanced-stage chronic lymphocytic leukaemia. The French Cooperative Group on CLL. *The Lancet* **347**, 1432–1438.

Keating, M., Manshouri, T., O'Brien S. *et al.* (2003). A high proportion of true complete remission can be obtained with a fludarabine, cyclophosphamide, rituximab combination (FCR) in chronic lymphocytic leukemia (abstract). *Proceedings of the American Society of Clinical Oncology* **22**, 569 (abstract 2289).

Keating, M. J., O'Brien, S., Lerner, S., Koller, C., Beran, M., Robertson, L. E., Freireich, E. J., Estey, E. & Kantarjian, H. (1998). Long-term follow-up of patients with chronic lymphocytic leukemia (CLL) receiving fludarabine regimens as initial therapy. *Blood* **92**, 1165–1171.

Kohl, U. L. *et al.* (1997). Synergistic cytoxicity using cyclophosphamide and nucleoside analogs (abstract). *Annals of Hematology* **74**, 75.

Leporrier, M., Chevret, S., Cazin, B., Boudjerra, N., Feugier, P., Desablens, B., Rapp, M. J., Jaubert, J., Autrand, C., Divine, M., Dreyfus, B., Maloum, K., Travade, P., Dighiero, G., Binet, J. L. & Chastang, C. (2001). Randomized comparison of fludarabine, CAP, and CHOP in 938 previously untreated stage B and C chronic lymphocytic leukemia patients. *Blood* **98**, 2319–2325.

Levy, V., Porcher, R., Delabarre, F., Leporrier, M., Cazin, B. & Chevret, S. (2001). Evaluating treatment strategies in chronic lymphocytic leukemia: use of quality-adjusted survival analysis. *Journal of Clinical Epidemiology* **54**, 747–754.

Lundin, J., Kimby, E., Bjorkholm, M., Broliden, P. A., Celsing, F., Hjalmar, V., Mollgard, L., Rebello, P., Hale, G., Waldmann, H., Mellstedt, H. & Osterborg, A. (2002). Phase II trial of subcutaneous anti-CD52 monoclonal antibody alemtuzumab (Campath-1H) as first-line treatment for patients with B-cell chronic lymphocytic leukemia (B-CLL). *Blood* **100**, 768–773.

O'Brien, S. M., Kantarjian, H., Thomas, D. A., Giles, F. J., Freireich, E. J., Cortes, J., Lerner, S. & Keating, M. J. (2001a). Rituximab dose-escalation trial in chronic lymphocytic leukemia. *Journal of Clinical Oncology* **19**, 2165–2170.

O'Brien, S. M., Kantarjian, H. M., Cortes, J., Beran, M., Koller, C. A., Giles, F. J., Lerner, S. & Keating, M. (2001b). Results of the fludarabine and cyclophosphamide combination regimen in chronic lymphocytic leukemia. *Journal of Clinical Oncology* **19**, 1414–1420.

Oscier, D., Orchard, J. A., Culligan, D., Cunningham, D., Johnson, S., Parker, A., Klein, M. & Gieschen, H. (2001). The bioavailability of oral fludarabine phosphate is unaffected by food. *Hematology Journal* **2**, 316–321.

Plunkett, W., Gandhi, V., Huang, P., Robertson, L. E., Yang, L. Y., Gregoire, V., Estey, E. & Keating, M. J. (1993). Fludarabine: pharmacokinetics, mechanisms of action, and rationales for combination therapies. *Seminars in Oncology* **20**, 2–12.

Rai, K., Byrd, J. C., Peterson, B. L. & Larson, R. A. (2002). A phase II trial of fludarabine followed by alemtuzumab (Campath 1H) in previously untreated chronic lymphocytic leukemia (CLL) patients with active disease : Cancer and Leukemia group B (CALGB) study 19901. *Blood* **100**, 205a.

Rai, K. R., Peterson, B. L., Appelbaum, F. R., Kolitz, J., Elias, L., Shepherd, L., Hines, J., Threatte, G. A., Larson, R. A., Cheson, B. D. & Schiffer, C. A. (2000). Fludarabine compared with chlorambucil as primary therapy for chronic lymphocytic leukemia. *New England Journal of Medicine* **343**, 1750–1757.

Rai, K. R., Sawitsky, A., Cronkite, E. P., Chanana, A. D., Levy, R. N. & Pasternack, B. S. (1975). Clinical staging of chronic lymphocytic leukemia. *Blood* **46**, 219–234.

Robak, T. (2001). Cladribine in the treatment of chronic lymphocytic leukemia. *Leukemia and Lymphoma* **40**, 551–564.

Robak, T., Blonski, J. Z., Kasznicki, M., Blasinska-Morawiec, M., Krykowski, E., Dmoszynska, A., Mrugala-Spiewak, H., Skotnicki, A. B., Nowak, W., Konopka, L., Ceglarek, B., Maj, S., Dwilewicz-Trojaczek, J., Hellmann, A., Urasinski, I., Zdziarska, B., Kotlarek-Haus, S., Potoczek, S. & Grieb, P. (2000). Cladribine with prednisone versus chlorambucil with prednisone as first-line therapy in chronic lymphocytic leukemia: report of a prospective, randomized, multicenter trial. *Blood* **96**, 2723–2729.

Robak, T., Blonski, J. Z., Kasznicki, M., Gora-Tybor, J., Dwilewicz-Trojaczek, J., Stella-Holowiecka, B. & Wolowiec, D. (2002). Cladribine combined with cyclophosphamide is highly effective in the treatment of chronic lymphocytic leukemia. *Hematology Journal* **3**, 244–250.

Rossi, J. F., van Hoof, A., de Boeck, K., Johnson, S., Bron, D., Foussard, C., Lister, T., Berthou, C., Kramer, M., Littlewood, T., Marcus, R., Deconinck, E., Montillo, M., Guibon, O. & Tollerfield, S. (2004). Efficacy and safety of oral fludarabine phosphate in previously untreated chronic lymphocytic leukemia. *Journal of Clinical Oncology* **22**(7), 1260–1267.

Schulz, H., Klein, S. K., Rehwald, U., Reiser, M., Hinke, A., Knauf, W. U., Aulitzky, W. E., Hensel, M., Herold, M., Huhn, D., Hallek, M., Diehl, V. & Engert, A. (2002). Phase 2 study of a combined immunochemotherapy using rituximab and fludarabine in patients with chronic lymphocytic leukemia. *Blood* **100**, 3115–3120.

Weiss, M. A., Maslak, P. G., Jurcic, J. G., Scheinberg, D. A., Aliff, T. B., Lamanna, N., Frankel, S. R., Kossman, S. E. & Horgan, D. (2003). Pentostatin and cyclophosphamide: an effective new regimen in previously treated patients with chronic lymphocytic leukemia. *Journal of Clinical Oncology* **21**, 1278–1284.

Chapter 7

Evidence and opinion for second-line intervention in chronic lymphocytic leukaemia

Stephen A. Johnson

Introduction

Clinical studies into the treatment of chronic lymphocytic leukaemia (B-CLL) have been undertaken for over half a century; the first active agents in the treatment of the disease were chlorambucil (Galton *et al.* 1955) and corticosteroids (Shaw *et al.* 1961). The evolution of approaches to the treatment of B-CLL has subsequently encompassed the use of alkylating agents, initially alone then in combination with anthracyclines and vinca alkaloids, then the era of purine analogues also initially evaluated as single agents then subsequently in combination therapies; recently the introduction of monoclonal antibodies heralds the era of immunotherapy or chemoimmunotherapy for B-CLL.

It has become apparent that B-CLL presents almost unique challenges for clinical researchers because the disease is heterogenous and patients may survive for many years with a significant proportion never requiring therapeutic interventions. Clinicians endeavouring to improve the outcome of patients who require treatment may often give several different types of therapy over the course of the disease and as a result the individual contribution of each successive drug or combination may be difficult to define. The exact level of activity of any treatment varies according to its place in the overall treatment strategy so that drugs which produce high rates of response when used as initial treatment may also make a substantial contribution to prolonging survival when given at later stages, especially if they are administered after less active agents.

Methods

The results of treatment trials in B-CLL published in peer-reviewed journals and as a part of the proceedings of the meetings of the American Society of Hematology, the American Society of Clinical Oncology and the International Workshop on Chronic Lymphocytic Leukaemia have been reviewed. Selection of studies for inclusion in this review has been made by the author on the basis of his personal evaluation and applying the criteria of the US Agency for Health Care Policy and Research to grade the evidence. The review is intended to supply guidance in principle concerning the choice of second-line therapy for B-CLL and as such is not intended to be a comprehensive source of all published studies in the field.

Results

It is self-evident that the results of second-line therapy for B-CLL will be affected both by the nature of the initial treatment and the response achieved by the prior therapy. Unfortunately the body of published data on which this review has drawn to make its recommendations contains very few studies in which the first-line therapy given to patients is documented in satisfactory detail. Many published studies of 'second-line treatment' include patients who have been exposed to a variety of 'first-line treatments' and entry criteria to these trials commonly permit more than one line of prior therapy. It is also sometimes difficult to distinguish within the patient populations between patients whose disease has merely relapsed after a satisfactory period of control and those who were refractory or unresponsive to their most recent prior treatment.

A body of historical data exists consisting largely of un-randomised studies from which an estimate of the activity of particular treatment modalities can be made. The contribution of randomised clinical trials is limited to a single phase III trial in previously treated patients with B-CLL, but several trials exist in which the subsequent treatment of patients randomised between first-line treatment options can be assessed by reviewing the outcome of crossing over from one arm to the other after treatment failure. Newer approaches to the treatment of patients with relapsed or refractory B-CLL are represented by phase II trials which may point to the treatment choices of the future. The conclusions which can be drawn from many of the published clinical experiences are limited by the variability of patient characteristics and the small size of the study populations.

For most patients with B-CLL, treatment is generally palliative in intent, the treatment options surrounding patients in whom high-dose therapy supported by autologous or allogeneic stem cells is planned will not be considered in this review. Patients who have relapsed B-CLL may be followed without therapy until they experience disease-related symptoms or progressive disease (associated with deterioration of blood counts, discomfort from lymphadenopathy or hepatosplenomegaly, recurrent infections or associated auto-immune phenomena) (Cheson et al. 1996). The indications for treatment of patients who have proved resistant to their first-line therapy are more straightforward as they are implicit in the initiation of the unsuccessful treatment already given, however this group of patients are likely to respond less well both because of the inherent difficulty of treating refractory disease and the likelihood of residual toxicity from the prior therapy.

The historical evidence for the efficacy of alkylator based treatment in patients requiring therapy is poorly documented as trials have not been conducted on the basis of planned second-line treatments. Patients who have experienced a response to an alkylating agent such as chlorambucil can often be successfully re-treated, however the quality of the response and its duration are less than that achieved with the initial treatment. A randomised study conducted by the Pethema Spanish Cooperative Group which included both first-line and previously treated patients (Montserrat *et al*. 1985) compared chlorambucil plus prednisone with a combination of cyclophosphamide, vincristine and prednisone (COP) and documented a significant advantage in overall response rate (ORR) for chlorambucil versus COP (59% versus 31%, $p < 0.01$). The study also highlighted the reduction in ORR in previously treated patients (the extent of prior treatment was not defined) compared with first-line therapy; although this was not significant for those treated with COP (33% versus 28%, *p*-value not significant) the fall in responses with chlorambucil was significant (71% versus 35%, $p < 0.05$) but numbers of evaluable patients were small in both groups (previously treated patients allocated to COP = 18, to chlorambucil/prednisone = 17).

Anthracycline-containing combinations consisting of cyclophosphamide, doxorubicin and prednisone with (CHOP) or without (CAP) vincristine have been extensively evaluated in studies of the initial therapy of B-CLL but once again the data for their use in previously treated patients is limited. A study conducted by a Danish group (Mork-Hansen & Anderson 1991) randomised patients between CHOP and chlorambucil plus prednisone; a total of 21 patients who were 'primarily or subsequently resistant to chlorambucil' were switched to CHOP and 15 were evaluable for response (ORR = 53%). Once again it is clear that numbers of evaluable patients are restricted as a basis for drawing conclusions about the efficacy of the combination in this setting, but at least the nature of the initial therapy is a consistent element.

Further evidence of the activity of anthracycline-based therapy in B-CLL comes from the only randomised phase III trial specifically designed to include previously treated patients which was conducted by an international collaborative group (French Cooperative Group on CLL *et al*. 1996). This study included both first-line patients and those with relapsed B-CLL 'pre-treated with chlorambucil and similar non-anthracycline or anthracenedione containing regimens for more than 6 months but less than 3 years' and randomised them between CAP and fludarabine. The ORR for CAP in pre-treated patients was 27%, significantly less than that achieved with fludarabine (48%, $p = 0.036$) and less than that achieved in the first-line population (60%); the median duration of response achieved with CAP was also shorter for the pre-treated group (179 days versus 208 days for untreated patients). Unfortunately no data concerning patients crossing over from one arm to the other after treatment failure is reported for this study.

The range of treatment options for B-CLL changed dramatically in 1988 with simultaneous reports of significant activity associated with the purine analogue fludarabine (Grever *et al*. 1988; Keating *et al*. 1988). Although the extent of prior treatment in the larger of these two cohorts (75 patients) of previously treated patients was variable, the ORR was 56% and a response rate of 50% was recorded for 32 patients who had received three or more lines of prior therapy (Keating *et al.* 1988). This level of response is similar to the ORR of 48% subsequently noted in the phase III trial already reviewed (French Cooperative Group on CLL *et al.* 1996) and in many other reports of the efficacy of fludarabine in previously treated patient populations (Keating *et al* 2000). A lower ORR of 32% was recorded by the National Cancer Institute as a result of access to fludarabine for heavily pre-treated patients through the Group C Protocol mechanism (Sorensen *et al.* 1997). A series of papers documenting the experience at the MD Anderson Cancer Center (Houston, Texas, USA) illustrates several important effects of fludarabine therapy; combination with prednisone does not affect the response rate, lack of initial response is associated with a very poor outcome, but re-treatment by fludarabine of patients achieving an initial response after relapse is associated with an excellent (ORR = 67%) chance of obtaining a further response (Keating *et al.* 1989, 1993, 1998). The evaluation of cladribine, another purine analogue has been slightly less extensive due to differences in opinion as to its correct schedule of administration. Levels of activity are however broadly similar based on results achieved by groups of investigators from the Scripps Institute (La Jolla, California, USA), Sweden and Poland among others. Approximately 55–85% of patients will achieve a response to cladribine as initial therapy (Saven *et al.* 1995; Juliusson *et al.* 1996; Robak *et al.* 2000a); as with other agents, the responses in previously treated patients vary according to the extent of prior treatment but in patients who have not been previously exposed to a purine analogue ORR of 44–67% can be achieved (Piro *et al.* 1988; Saven *et al.* 1991; Juliusson & Liliemark 1993; Robak *et al.* 2000a). As with fludarabine, it is possible to achieve further responses with cladribine in patients who have had reasonable remissions with cladribine as first-line therapy (Juliusson & Liliemark 1994, 1996).

There are four randomised phase III studies which compare purine analogue therapy with alkylator based treatments for first-line therapy and which therefore offer the opportunity to examine a well characterised cohort of patients who cross-over to alternative therapy after failure of the treatment to which they were initially allocated. The US Intergroup Study compared fludarabine (170 patients) with pulsed chlorambucil (181 patients) (Rai *et al.* 2000). Of the 63 patients who did not respond to fludarabine, 29 were crossed over to chlorambucil but only 2 (7%) achieved a response; traffic in the opposite direction involved 79 of the 114 patients who did not respond to chlorambucil and 36 (43%) of these responded to fludarabine achieving an ORR in the range predicted from unrandomised studies (56% in Keating *et al* (1988)) and the randomised phase III trial of previously treated patients (48% in French Cooperative Group on CLL *et al.* 1996). A separate study conducted by the French Collaborative Group (Leporrier *et al.* 2001) randomised patients between fludarabine and two anthracycline based combinations (CAP or CHOP); responses for the 97 patients crossing over to fludarabine were good (42%) but significant efficacy was also seen in the smaller number of patients failing fludarabine and receiving CHOP (12/31, ORR 38.7%). The final trial which contributed data to this enquiry randomised patients between cladribine and chlorambucil (prednisone in both arms) (Robak *et al.* 2000b); there is again evidence of greater benefit to patients who fail chlorambucil and cross-over to cladribine (29/43, ORR = 67%) than in the other direction (7/26, ORR = 27%). In this study CHOP was recommended as the third-line treatment choice achieving similar levels of response irrespective of the initial randomisation (cladribine *n* = 15, ORR 20%; chlorambucil *n* = 11, ORR 27%) indicating that the sequence of treatment choices is not relevant to the outcome at this stage. The studies considered above are summarised in Table 7.1.

Further evidence on the subsequent clinical course of patients who have received a purine analogue as their initial therapy is inevitably somewhat more recent. There has been a longstanding assumption that the activity of fludarabine and cladribine is broadly equivalent in the treatment of B-CLL and that changing from one to the other is unlikely to be beneficial in patients with evidence of resistance. A small case series which reported benefit from cladribine therapy in 3 patients who were refractory to fludarabine (Juliusson *et al.* 1992) was not confirmed by the experience of other investigators but a recent study sponsored by the Cancer and Leukaemia Group B (Byrd *et al.* 2003) has achieved responses in 9 out of 28 patients (ORR 32%), challenging previous assumptions.

Phase II studies reported in the purine analogue era must be carefully sorted to distinguish whether prior treatment has included fludarabine or cladribine and also to identify whether patients were included at untested relapse or were resistant to the last treatment they received (summarised in Table 7.2). For those patients who have not been exposed to purine analogues and who have non-resistant disease or late (>12 months) relapse, response rates of 42–59% can be achieved with fludarabine ± prednisone (Keating *et al* 1988, 1989, 2000, 2002b; French Cooperative Group on CLL *et al.* 1996; Leporrier *et al.* 2001; Rai *et al.* 2000) and of 44–67% with cladribine ± prednisone (Robak *et al.* 2000a; Piro *et al.* 1988; Saven *et al.* 1991; Juliusson & Liliemark 1993). When purine analogues are administered in combination with other agents, reported responses are increased although studies are smaller; examples include studies of fludarabine in combination with epirubicin (*n* = 25, ORR 62%) (Rummel *et al.* 1999) or cyclophosphamide (n=20, ORR 85%) (O'Brien 2001) and also similar results reported by the German Collaborative Group (*n* = 18, ORR 94%) (Hallek *et al.* 2001); efficacy has also been demonstrated for the combination of fludarabine with cyclophosphamide and mitozantrone (ORR = 72%) (Bosch *et al.* 2002).

Data on populations of patients who are clearly resistant to prior non-purine analogue based therapy are more difficult to extract from the published studies, but the ORR to fludarabine in this setting is reduced to 38% (Keating *et al.* 1993).

Turning to the patient population who have been exposed to purine analogues and undergone late relapse, the response rate for re-treatment with fludarabine alone is 68% (Keating *et al.* 1998; 2002b); the results for cladribine are probably similar but less well documented. Efficacy of combinations in this setting is similar for fludarabine and doxorubicin ($n = 25$, ORR = 55%) (Robertson *et al.* 1995) but much better with fludarabine plus cyclophosphamide ($n = 46$, ORR = 80%) (O'Brien *et al.* 2001). Those patients who have received fludarabine and were resistant to their last treatment predictably do less well (Keating *et al.* 1998, 2002b) but responses can be achieved with fludarabine + doxorubicin ($n = 5$, ORR = 40%) (Robertson *et al.* 1995) and fludarabine + cyclophosphamide ($n = 28$, ORR = 39%) (O'Brien *et al.* 2001) and fludarabine + cyclophosphamide + mitozantrone (ORR = 34%) (Bosch *et al.* 2002).

Although it is widely used there is little published data on the efficacy of high dose methylprednisolone (HDMP). A pilot study reported responses in 6 out of 11 patients with advanced refractory B-CLL (ORR = 55%), but the extent of prior treatment was variable and only a proportion of patients in the study had been exposed to purine analogues (Thornton *et al.* 1999).

Two therapeutic monoclonal antibodies have undergone reasonably extensive evaluation in the treatment of B-CLL. Rituximab (anti-CD20) has considerable activity against other B-cell malignancies but response rates to its use as a single agent in previously treated patients with B-CLL are poor. In a study of conventional treatment (375 mg/m^2/week) for 4 weeks, 7 out of 28 patients (25%) achieved a partial response (Huhn *et al.* 2002) but even with very high doses (up to six times the standard dose) using a weekly schedule all the responses are partial; 9/16 (56%) of patients with disease sensitive to fludarabine responded compared with 4/20 (20%) who were previously resistant (O'Brien 2001). Using a three times weekly schedule evidence of some efficacy was found in non-resistant patients ($n = 10$, ORR = 30%) and in fludarabine-refractory patients ($n = 17$, ORR = 41%) (Byrd *et al.* 2001).

Suggestions that rituximab may have a synergistic action with cytotoxic chemotherapy are supported by a study which administered rituximab with fludarabine to patients with non-resistant, non-purine analogue exposed disease and achieved a high response rate ($n = 11$, ORR = 90%) (Schulz *et al.* 2002). An extensive experience is being accumulated at the MD Anderson Cancer Center of the combination of fludarabine, cyclophosphamide and rituximab, which appears to be highly active in all settings; responses are obtained in resistant non-fludarabine exposed patients ($n = 15$, ORR = 66%), fludarabine sensitive patients ($n = 60$, ORR = 78%) and fludarabine-resistant patients ($n = 27$, ORR = 59%) (Manero 2002).

Alemtuzumab (anti-CD52) has significant activity in the treatment of B-CLL producing responses in refractory non-purine analogue treated patients ($n = 29$, ORR = 42%) (Osterborg *et al.* 1997) and in patients refractory to fludarabine ($n = 92$, ORR = 33%) (Keating *et al.* 2002a) ($n = 24$, ORR = 33%) (Rai *et al.* 2002). The limitations to the use of alemtuzumab relate to toxicity secondary to profound immunosuppression and its relatively poor activity in sites of bulky disease.

Discussion

It is possible to grade and assess the evidence presented above to provide advice for clinicians treating patients in the UK in 2003. Many patients will be entered into the current national trial involving randomisation between chlorambucil, fludarabine and fludarabine plus cyclophosphamide, while a number who are unsuitable for a study which might result in purine analogue therapy will receive chlorambucil without study entry. The guidance below is drawn from the guidelines of the British Committee for Standards in Haematology. The possibilities for second-line therapy and subsequent treatment options are therefore:

1. Patients who relapse after an initial response to low dose chlorambucil outside of a trial setting may be treated with a further course of chlorambucil. Grade B recommendation: level IIb evidence;
2. Patients refractory to low dose chlorambucil should be treated with fludarabine. CHOP is an alternative treatment for patients unsuitable for fludarabine. Grade B recommendation: level IIb evidence.
3. Patients who develop progressive disease over one year since receiving fludarabine and whose CLL responded to fludarabine initially, may be treated again with fludarabine alone. Grade B recommendation: level IIb evidence.
4. Patients who develop progressive disease within one year of previous fludarabine therapy may be treated with a combination of fludarabine and cyclophosphamide. Grade B recommendation: level IIb evidence.
5. Patients who are refractory or become resistant to fludarabine currently have a poor prognosis. Therapeutic options include the following:
    (a) High dose methylprednisolone. Grade B recommendation: level III evidence.
    (b) Alemtuzumab. Grade B recommendation: level IIb evidence.
    (c) Rituximab monotherapy is not recommended. Grade C recommendation: level 2b evidence.
    (d) Rituximab + fludarabine ± cyclophosphamide may be effective. Grade B recommendation: level 2b evidence.
6. Autologous or allogeneic transplantation may be considered in suitable patients.

Acknowledgements

I thank Michael Keating for his inspiration and Chris Fegan who collaborated in producing the guidelines to treatment.

Table 7.1 CLL Therapy: first- and second-line response rates

	First line (%)	Second line (%)	Salvage
Chlorambucil/prednisone	71	35	
COP	33	28	
CAP	60	27	
CHOP	72	53	20–27
Fludarabine	71–78	42–59	32
Cladribine	55–85	44–67	

Table 7.2 CLL Therapy: response rate by prior treatment and response

	No prior purine analogue		Prior purine analogues	
	Resistant or early relapse (%)	Non-resistant or late relapse (%)	Resistant or early relapse (%)	Non-resistant or late relapse (%)
Fludarabine ± prednisone	37	44–59	0	68
Fludarabine + epirubicin or doxorubicin		62	40	55
Fludarabine + cyclophosphamide		85–94	39	80
Fludarabine + cyclophosphamide + mitozantrone	34	72		
Cladribine ± prednisone		44–67	32	
High dose methylpredisone	20		40	
Rituximab (dose esc)			41 (20)	30 (56)
Fludarabine + rituximab		90		
Fludarabine + cyclophosphamide + rituximab	66		59	78
Alemtuzumab	42		33	

References

Bosch, F., Ferrer, A., Lopez-Guillermo, A. *et al.* (2002). Fludarabine, cyclophosphamide and mitoxantrone in the treatment of resistant or relapsed chronic lymphocytic leukaemia. *British Journal of Haematology* **119**, 976–984.

Byrd, J. C., Murphy, T., Howard, R. S. *et al.* (2001). Rituximab using a twice weekly dosing schedule in B-cell chronic lymphocytic leukemia and small lymphocytic lymphoma demonstrates clinical activity and acceptable toxicity. *Journal of Clinical Oncology* **19**, 2153–2164.

Byrd, J.C., Peterson, B., Piro, L. *et al.* (2003). A phase II study of cladribine treatment for fludarabine refractory B-cell chronic lymphocytic leukemia: results from CALGB study 9211. *Leukemia* **17**, 323–327.

Cheson, B. D., Bennett, J. M., Grever, M. *et al.* (1996). National Cancer Institute-sponsored working group guidelines for chronic lymphocytic leukemia: revised guidelines for diagnosis and treatment. *Blood* **87**, 4990–4997.

French Cooperative Group on CLL, Johnson, S., Smith, A. G. *et al.* (1996). Multicentre prospective randomised trial of fludarabine versus cyclophosphamide, doxorubicin and prednisone (CAP) for treatment of advanced stage chronic lymphocytic leukaemia. *The Lancet* **347**, 1432–1438.

Galton, D. A. G., Israels, L. G., Nabarro, J. D. N. *et al.* (1955). Clinical trials of p(di-2-chloroethylamino)-phenylbutyric acid (CD 1348) in malignant lymphoma. *British Medical Journal* **2**, 1172–1176.

Grever, M. R., Kopecky, K. J., Coltman, C. A. *et al.* (1988). Fludarabine monophosphate: a potentially useful agent in chronic lymphocytic leukaemia. *Nouvelle Revue Francaise d'Hematologie* **30**, 457–459.

Hallek, M., Schmitt, B., Wilhelm, M. *et al.* (2001). Fludarabine plus cyclophosphamide is an efficient treatment for advanced chronic lymphocytic leukaemia (CLL): results of a phase II study of the German CLL Study Group. *British Journal of Haematology* **114**, 342–348.

Huhn, D., von Schilling, C., Wilhelm, M. *et al.* (2002). Rituximab therapy of patients with B-cell chronic lymphocytic leukemia. *Blood* **98**, 1326–1331.

Juliusson, G., Christiansen, I., Mork-Hansen, M. *et al.* (1996). Oral cladribine as primary therapy for patients with B-cell chronic lymphocytic leukaemia. *Journal of Clinical Oncology* **14**, 2160–2166.

Juliusson, G., Elmhorn-Rosenborg, A. & Liliemark, J. (1992). Response to chlorodeoxyadenosine in patients with B-cell chronic lymphocytic leukemia resistant to fludarabine. *New England Journal of Medicine* **327**, 1056–1061.

Juliusson, G. & Liliemark, J. (1993). High complete remission rate from 2-chloro-2'-deoxyadenosine in previously treated patients with B-cell chronic lymphocytic leukaemia: response predicted by rapid decrease of blood lymphocyte count. *Journal of Clinical Oncology* **11**, 679–689.

Juliusson, G. & Liliemark, J. (1994). Retreatment of chronic lymphocytic leukaemia with 2-chlorodeoxyadenosine (CdA) at relapse following CdA-induced remission: no acquired resistance. *Leukemia & Lymphoma* **13**, 75–80.

Juliusson, G. & Liliemark, J. (1996). Long-term survival following cladribine (2-chlorodeoxyadenosine) therapy in previously treated patients with chronic lymphocytic leukaemia. *Annals of Oncology* **7**, 373–379.

Keating, M. J., Flinn, I., Jain, V. *et al.* (2002a). Therapeutic role of alemtuzumab (Campath 1-H) in patients who have failed fludarabine: results of a large international study. *Blood* **99**, 3554–3561.

Keating, M. J., Kantarjian, H., Talpaz, M. *et al.* (1988). Fludarabine therapy in chronic lymphocytic leukaemia (CLL). *Nouvelle Revue Francaise d'Hematologie* **30**, 461–466.

Keating, M. J., Kantarjian, H., Talpaz, M. *et al.* (1989). Fludarabine: a new agent with major activity against chronic lymphocytic leukaemia. *Blood* **74**, 19–25.

Keating, M. J., O'Brien, S., Kantarjian, H. *et al.* (1993). Long-term follow-up of patients with chronic lymphocytic leukaemia (CLL) treated with fludarabine as a single agent. *Blood* **81**, 2878–2884.

Keating, M. J., O'Brien, S., Kontoyiannis, D. *et al.* (2002b). Results of first salvage therapy for patients refractory to a fludarabine regimen in chronic lymphocytic leukaemia. *Leukemia and Lymphoma* **43**, 1755–1762.

Keating, M. J., O'Brien, S., Lerner, S. *et al.* (1998) Long-term follow-up of patients with chronic lymphocytic leukaemia (CLL) receiving fludarabine regimens as initial therapy. *Blood* **92**, 1165–1171.

Keating, M. J., Smith, T. L., Lerner, S *et al.* (2000) Prediction of prognosis following fludarabine used as secondary therapy for chronic lymphocytic leukaemia. *Leukemia & Lymphoma* **37**, 71–85.

Leporrier, M., Chevret, S., Cazin, B. *et al.* (2001). Randomised comparison of fludarabine, CAP and CHOP in 938 previously untreated stage B and C chronic lymphocytic leukaemia patients. *Blood* **98**, 2319–2325.

Manero, G. G., O'Brien, S., Cortes, J. *et al.* (2002). Update of results for the combination of fludarabine, cyclophosphamide and rituximab for previously treated patients with chronic lymphocytic leukaemia (CLL). *Blood* **98**, 633a (abstract 2650).

Montserrat, E., Alcala, A., Parody, R. *et al.* (1985). Treatment of chronic lymphocytic leukaemia in advanced stages: a randomised trial comparing chlorambucil plus prednisone versus cyclophosphamide, vincristine and prednisone. *Cancer* **56**, 2369–2375.

Mork-Hansen, M. & Anderson, E. (1991). CHOP versus chlorambucil + prednisone in chronic lymphocytic leukaemia. *Leukemia & Lymphoma* **5** (Suppl.), 97–100.

O'Brien, S. M., Kantarjian, H. M., Cortes, J. *et al.* (2001). Results of the fludarabine and cyclophosphamide combination regimen in chronic lymphocytic leukemia. *Journal of Clinical Oncology* **19**, 1414–1420.

O'Brien, S. M., Kantarjian, H., Thomas, D. A. *et al.* (2001). Rituximab dose-escalation trial in chronic lymphocytic leukemia. *Journal of Clinical Oncology* **19**, 2165–2170.

Osterborg, A., Dyer, M. J. S., Bunjes, D. *et al.* (1997). Phase II multicenter study of human CD52 antibody in previously treated chronic lymphocytic leukemia. European Group of CAMPATH-1H treatment in chronic lymphocytic leukemia. *Journal of Clinical Oncology* **15**, 1567–1574.

Piro, L. D., Carrera, C.J., Beutler, E. *et al.* (1988). 2-chlorodeoxyadenosine: an effective new agent for the treatment of chronic lymphocytic leukemia. *Blood* **72**, 1069–1073.

Rai, K. R., Freter, C. E., Mercier, M. R. *et al.* (2002). Alemtuzumab in previously treated chronic lymphocytic leukaemia in patients who also had received fludarabine. *Journal of Clinical Oncology* **18**, 3891–3897.

Rai, K. R., Peterson, B. L., Appelbaum, F. R. *et al.* (2000). Fludarabine compared with chlorambucil a primary therapy for chronic lymphocytic leukaemia. *New England Journal of Medicine* **343**, 1750–1757.

Robak, T., Blonski, J. Z., Kasznicki, M. *et al.* (2000a). Cladribine with or without prednisone in the treatment of previously treated and untreated B-cell chronic lymphocytic leukaemia – updated results of the multicentre study of 378 patients. *British Journal of Haematology* **108**, 357–368.

Robak, T., Blonski, J. Z., Kasznicki, M. *et al.* (2000b). Cladribine with prednisone versus chlorambucil with prednisone as first-line therapy in chronic lymphocytic leukemia: report of a prospective, randomized, multicenter trial. *Blood* **96**, 2723–2729.

Robertson, L. E., O'Brien, S., Kantarjian, H (1995). Fludarabine plus doxorubicin in previously treated chronic lymphocytic leukaemia. *Leukemia* **9**, 943–945.

Rummel, M. J., Kafer, G., Pfreundschuh, M. *et al.* (1999). Fludarabine and epirubicin in the treatment of chronic lymphocytic leukaemia: a German Multicentre phase II study. *Annals of Oncology* **10**, 183–188.

Saven, A., Carrera, C. J., Carson, D. A. *et al.* (1991). 2-chlorodeoxyadenosine treatment of refractory chronic lymphocytic leukaemia. *Leukemia & Lymphoma* **5** (Suppl.), 133–138.

Saven, A., Lemon, R. H., Kosty, M. *et al.* (1995). 2-chlorodeoxyadenosine activity in patients with untreated chronic lymphocytic leukaemia. *Journal of Clinical Oncology* **14**, 2160–2166.

Schulz, H., Klein, S. K., Rehwald, U. *et al.* (2002). Phase 2 study of a combined immunochemotherapy using rituximab and fludarabine in patients with chronic lymphocytic leukemia. *Blood* **100**, 3115–3120.

Shaw, R. K., Boggs, D. R., Silberman, H. R. *et al.* (1961). A study of prednisone therapy in chronic lymphatic leukaemia. *Blood* **17**, 182–189.

Sorensen, J. M., Vena, D. A., Fallavollita, A. *et al.* (1997). Treatment of refractory chronic lymphocytic leukaemia with fludarabine phosphate via the Group C Protocol mechanism of the National Cancer Institute: five-year follow-up report. *Journal of Clinical Oncology* **15**, 458–465.

Thornton, P. D., Hamblin, M., Treleaven, J. G. *et al.* (1999). High dose methylprednisolone in refractory chronic lymphocytic leukemia. *Leukemia & Lymphoma* **34**, 167–170.

PART 3

Evidence and opinion for medical intervention – II

Chapter 8

Stem-cell transplantation for chronic lymphocytic leukaemia

Donald W. Milligan

Introduction

Most patients with chronic lymphocytic leukaemia (CLL) are elderly, and in older patients the increased morbidity and mortality of high-dose chemo-radiotherapy with allogeneic or autologous stem-cell rescue do not justify this approach. About 20% of patients are younger than 65. CLL in young adults has no major distinctive features, the prognostic factors are the same as those in older patients and median survival is less than three years for young patients with advanced CLL (Mauro *et al.* 1999). In these younger patients it may well be justifiable to consider a more aggressive approach when standard treatment with alkylating agents or purine analogues offers a poor outlook. To date the only potentially curative therapy for CLL is by autologous or allogeneic transplantation. The risks and benefits vary considerably between the types of treatment available from a transplant-related mortality of less than 5% for the current practice of autologous transplantation to over 40% for some allogeneic transplants. In these circumstances it is critical that a full understanding is obtained from patients about the degree of risk they wish to be exposed to (including the risks of debilitating graft versus host disease) balanced against the potential gain of the treatment. There are a large number of uncertainties concerning the optimum transplant treatment options for patients with CLL and where possible patients should be enrolled into randomised clinical trials or treated as part of a clinical research protocol.

Autologous transplantation

Autologous transplantation is based on the premise that for some chemotherapeutic regimens there is a dose effect and that superior anti-tumour efficacy can be achieved by dose escalation. There is some logic to this in CLL since conventional dose escalation results in increased response rates (Gale and Montserrat, 1993). There have been no randomised studies of autologous transplantation versus standard chemotherapy in CLL. The first published studies of autografting came from Boston (Rabinowe *et al.* 1993) and subsequently extended (Gribben *et al.* 1998). In this series patients with CLL were transplanted after achievement of a good response to prior (unspecified) chemotherapy. The conditioning regimen was cyclophosphamide and

TBI and the stem-cell source was bone marrow purged *in vivo* with a cocktail of monoclonal antibodies (B5, anti-CD10 and anti-CD20). The procedure-related mortality was 10% but the most striking observation was that at four years the disease-free survival was 63% and the overall survival was 85%. Most achieved a complete clinical response after the autograft procedure, and over 50% were IgH polymerase chain reaction (PCR) negative using sequence specific oligonucleotide probes (Provan *et al.* 1996). In addition, the achievement of successful purging of the marrow, as tested by IgH PCR, was associated with a better outlook. It remains unclear if this result is due to a lower burden of marrow disease in those patients whose marrow harvest became PCR negative compared with those who did not.

Other studies of autografting in CLL have produced less impressive results. In a small study from the M. D. Anderson Center, Houston, Texas, USA (Khouri *et al.* 1994) 7 of 11 patients achieved a complete response (CR) after autografting but these were short-lived and two patients died of transplant-related complications. Larger series have been reported in abstract form (Montserrat *et al.* 1999; Horowitz *et al.* 1999; Scimé *et al* 1998; Dreger *et al.* 2000b; Forsyth *et al.* 2000). The UK MRC have recently reported (Milligan *et al.* 2004) the results of the UK CLL Pilot Study in which 65 patients were autografted with a five year overall and disease-free survival of 78% (CI 57–98%) and 52% (CI 33–70%), respectively. The European Bone Marrow Transplant Group (EBMT) (Dreger *et al.* 2000b) reported 321 patients with a median age of 51 years. Seventy-eight per cent of patients received peripheral blood grafts; B-cell purging, either by CD34 selection or the use of anti-B-cell monoclonals, was attempted in about half. The transplant-related mortality was 6%; 83% of patients were alive at two years. Favourable prognostic indicators were complete remission at the time of transplant and the use of total body irradiation (TBI) in the conditioning schedule. Subsequent reviews have shown that the transplant-related mortality ranges from 4% to 10%, and that 65–94% of patients are alive at four years from transplantation (Van Besien *et al.* 2001; Dreger and Montserrat 2002). The outcome after autologous transplantation appears to be improved in patients with mutated IgV_H genes (Ritgen *et al.* 2003), and patients with del11q23 have a lower chance of achieving a minimal residual disease (MRD)-negative state post-autograft (Stilgenbauer *et al.* 2000). There is no evidence to suggest that autologous transplantation in CLL is curative, based on the lack of plateau in survival curves and the high risk of clinical relapse in patients who either fail to achieve a molecular CR or who develop molecular disease. In the absence of a randomised trial it remains unclear whether an autograft delivers benefit in terms of either survival or freedom from disease. A matched pair analysis comparing two cohorts of patients in Germany has attempted to answer this question (Dreger *et al.* 2002). This has shown an apparent survival advantage in favour of the autografted patients although, of course, such retrospective analyses must be treated with caution.

Patient selection bias

Most studies of autografting in CLL report data either from the time of stem-cell mobilisation or from the transplant date. This introduces a substantial bias because it is impossible to discern from the information presented how many patients failed to receive the autograft either because they did not achieve an adequate response to initial chemotherapy or because it proved impossible to collect adequate stem cells. Thus the true impact of an autograft strategy on the whole CLL population is difficult to ascertain. Some of these deficiencies have been addressed in the MRC CLL Pilot Study (Milligan *et al.* 2004) where patients were registered at the start of induction treatment. Of 100 patients entered, only about 50% received a transplant because of a poor response to chemotherapy or inadequate stem-cell mobilisation. Similar results have been reported from elsewhere. In a German study (Dreger and Schmitz 1997), 18 patients received one or two cycles of dexa-BEAM followed by a B-cell-depleted bone marrow or stem-cell harvest, and 13 of the patients proceeded to autograft. A French group (Sutton *et al.* 1998) enrolled 20 patients with advanced or refractory CLL treated with ESHAP followed by autologous transplantation. Only 13 patients achieved a satisfactory response to the induction schedule. Stem-cell mobilisation was attempted in 12 and was successful in 8. Only eight patients proceeded to an autograft.

Stem-cell mobilisation in CLL

The use of peripheral blood stem cells has rapidly superseded bone marrow as a source of marrow re-populating cells in many areas. This is because larger stem-cell doses can be achieved and these are associated with faster engraftment, reduced length of stay and a reduction in transplant-related costs. Transplant-related mortality has also fallen although it is less clear whether this is related to better case selection or the faster engraftment. Difficulty with stem-cell harvesting is a common problem in CLL. The reasons for this are probably twofold: CLL is associated with a heavy bone marrow burden of disease and is treated with alkylating agents or fludarabine, which may damage the stem-cell compartment. The relative contribution of these components is difficult to dissect. Fludarabine is the most potent agent in the treatment of CLL (Rai *et al.* 2000) and the effective elimination of bone marrow infiltration may improve the ability to mobilise stem cells (Itala *et al.* 1997). Results from the EBMT (Michallet *et al.* 2000) showed that treatment with more than six cycles of treatment with fludarabine was associated with improved stem-cell mobilisation, as was a delay of more than two months to mobilisation following the last cycle of treatment. However, these findings are contradicted in reports in indolent lymphoid malignancy (Ketterer *et al.* 1998; Sala *et al.* 1998; Flinn *et al.* 2000) and acute myeloid leukaemia (Visani et al. 1999) where prior therapy with fludarabine impaired the ability to mobilise stem cells. It is probable that two competing influences are at play here and further studies are needed to define the optimal cytoreductive and mobilisation regimens in CLL.

Peripheral blood or bone marrow purging

At the time of bone marrow or peripheral blood stem-cell harvest, CLL cells are always detectable by sensitive techniques and it is thus tempting to hope that the outlook might be improved by 'purging' the harvest by CD34 selection or negative selection using anti-B-cell antibodies. There have been no randomised studies of the impact of this strategy on the outcome, and there are several problems. Because of the difficulty in obtaining large numbers of stem cells and the cell loss associated with many of the purging methods, purging cannot always be performed. This was true in approximately 50% of the cases in the MRC Pilot Study (Milligan *et al.* 2004). Purging also remains inefficient at removing CLL cells; in the Boston series (Provan *et al.* 1996) 11 of 21 patients had detectable disease in the harvest after exposure to a cocktail of three B-cell monoclonal antibodies. The German group (Dreger *et al.* 1998) used either CD34 selection or negative selection with B-cell monoclonals but found that although 9 of 11 harvests were negative by flow cytometry, only three were negative using the more sensitive technique of PCR for IgH re-arrangements. Although it has been reported that successful clearance of CLL cells is associated with a reduced relapse risk (Provan *et al.* 1996), it is by no means clear that the purging was the important factor; it remains possible that the patients in whom the harvest was successfully eradicated had a lower burden of disease than those in whom the harvest remained CLL positive. The development of a molecular CR post-transplant is often associated, in parallel with myeloma, with infusion of cells expressing the CLL phenotype at autograft (Barlogie *et al.* 1987; Morgan *et al.* 2001). It is likely given the long molecular remissions that can, on occasion, be obtained after infusion of apparent CLL cells that only a proportion of the infused cells have clonogenic potential. In the MRC CLL Pilot Study, CD34 selection was not associated with any reduction of relapse risk (Morgan *et al.* 2001). From the above it is difficult to know if CLL purging as currently practised has any impact on the course of the disease. It is therefore recommended that purging strategies are undertaken only as part of carefully constructed clinical trials.

Using standard cytoreductive therapy, it is rare for patients to become PCR negative for CLL although 30% may achieve a complete remission as defined by the NCI criteria (Rai *et al.* 2000). The advent of the humanised monoclonal antibodies rituximab (anti CD20) or Campath 1H (anti CD52) alone or combined with chemotherapy has changed this, and a proportion of patients may now be rendered PCR negative by using *in vivo* purging (Rai *et al.* 2000; Kennedy *et al.* 2000; Keating *et al.* 2000). The relevance of this to the outcome of autologous transplantation has not yet been established. *In vivo* purging has principally been used to allow previously chemoresistant patients to achieve a CR or partial response and to then progress to an autograft (Forsyth *et al.* 2000). Formal studies are required to demonstrate whether the results of autotransplantation will be improved by the development of a molecular CR pre-transplant.

Conditioning regimens

Eradication of residual tumour can be achieved either with total body irradiation and chemotherapy (usually TBI/cyclophosphamide) or chemotherapy alone. A multivariate retrospective analysis by the EBMT (Dreger *et al.* 2000a) suggests that TBI/cyclophosphamide is associated with a reduced relapse risk and superior overall survival. The recent UK MRC study has, however, highlighted a worrying incidence of secondary leukaemia after the use of cyclophosphamide and TBI (Milligan *et al.* 2004) and although this has not been confirmed by others it is difficult in the light of current knowledge to be definitive about conditioning regimens.

Quality of life

There are no published data of quality of life after autologous transplantation in CLL compared with other treatments. Because of the considerable morbidity associated with this procedure this is a deficiency that future studies will seek to correct. A carefully conducted retrospective matched pair analysis has suggested that autografting may be associated with a survival advantage compared with standard treatment (Dreger *et al.* 2002) but this study can be criticised because of the different periods of treatment in the two different cohorts. A full understanding of the value or otherwise of autografting in CLL will only be established in the context of randomised clinical trials such as the MRC CLL 5 trial. Although autografting is associated with molecular CRs in 70% of patients, these are not usually durable and it is not known whether the procedure will translate into improved overall survival or improved quality of life. Because of this, it is recommended that stem-cell autografts in CLL be undertaken as part of a clinical research protocol, ideally in a randomised prospective trial.

Allografting in chronic lymphocytic leukaemia
Standard allografts

Allogeneic transplantation is unhampered by the difficulties of mobilising stem cells or of the risk of infusing clonogenic tumour cells. Allo-transplantation is, however, associated with substantial morbidity and mortality caused by organ failure due to conditioning therapy, acute and chronic graft versus host disease and the risks of infection. Patients with CLL are generally older than most patients undergoing allogeneic transplants, and these risks are consequently greater. An early study of patients reported to the International Bone Marrow Transplant Registry (IBMTR) and EBMT of 54 patients (Michallet *et al.* 1996) demonstrated that allogeneic transplantation was feasible and remission was achieved in 38 patients. The non-relapse mortality was 46% and the three-year probability of survival was 46% (32–60%). In a subsequent EBMT survey examining the outcome of 380 transplanted patients, the average age of those receiving allogeneic transplants in CLL was 44 years compared with 50 years for autotransplants (Michallet *et al.* 1999). In this retrospective study there was a very significant difference in the transplant-related mortality for allografting versus autografting (50% versus 13%), although the allograft recipients in general had more advanced disease at the time of transplant. In another single centre study (Pavletic *et al.* 2000), 23 patients underwent a conventional allotransplant from a related (20) or unrelated (3) donor. Fourteen patients had chemo-refractory disease. Eighty-seven per cent achieved a CR but the incidence of grade II–IV graft-versus-host disease (GVHD) was 54%. Eight patients died of transplant-related complications but 61% of patients were alive and disease free at a median of 26 months. A report from the IBMTR (Horowitz *et al.* 2000) identified 325 transplanted patients (242 allograft; 83 autograft). The three-year survival probability was 45% for allografted patients and 87% for autografts.

These reports suggest that allografting can be an effective treatment for some patients with CLL and that achievement of a molecular complete remission is more likely than after autografting (Esteve *et al.* 2001). However, compared with allografting, patients receiving an autograft fare better, at least initially, because of the unacceptably high transplant-related mortality of conventional allograft regimens in CLL. There will be some settings where it is not possible to perform an autograft, for instance where it has not been possible to harvest stem cells or where there is disease resistance. In these circumstances an allograft may offer some younger patients with high-risk disease the potential for cure, but the potential gains have to be balanced against the considerable early mortality. The observation that patients with evidence of chronic lymphocytic leukaemia after transplant can eradicate this following donor lymphocyte infusions strongly suggests that the long-term disease-free survival achievable after allogeneic transplantation is immunologically mediated (Ritgen *et al.* 2002). These data, together with the high treatment-related mortality associated with standard allogeneic transplantation, have provided the impetus for studies using low-intensity conditioning regimens.

Low-intensity allografts

One of the potential advantages of allografting is the harnessing of a graft versus tumour effect. That this can occur in CLL has been demonstrated by the elimination of leukaemia after transplant either by the cessation of immunosuppressive therapy or by the use of donor lymphocyte infusions (Jarque *et al.* 1993; Mehta *et al.* 1996; Rondon *et al* 1996; Mattsson *et al.* 2000). In recent years there has been an appreciation that this graft versus leukaemia effect can be harnessed by using non-myeloablative regimens which may be associated with a reduced early mortality due to transplant complications. These transplants are usually conditioned with regimens containing fludarabine as an immunosuppressive treatment or low dose TBI. Initial reports from M D Anderson Cancer Centre, Houston suggested that the GVHD risks after such transplants were low, postulating that this was because of the effect of fludarabine treatment on host dendritic cells which are thought to be important for the generation of GVHD (Khouri *et al.* 1997). Only limited numbers of transplants in CLL have been reported using low intensity or 'mini' transplants (Khouri *et al.* 1998; Cull *et al* 2000) The early optimism of this approach has been tempered by the realisation that the non-relapse mortality remains high in vulnerable groups of older patients with advanced disease and that disabling graft versus host disease can result in considerable reduction in quality of life (Giralt *et al.* 2001). The risks of graft versus host disease may be reduced by the use of T-cell depletion strategies at the time of transplant. The anti-CD52 antibody Campath 1H has been associated with a very low risk of GVHD after non-myeloablative transplants (Cull *et al.* 2000; Kottaridis *et al.* 2000), although there is an increased risk of post-transplant infections in these patients because of reduced donor T-cell recovery. A recent review of 77 patients in Europe undergoing a low-intensity allogeneic transplant for CLL has revealed considerable heterogeneity in both conditioning schedules and GVHD prophylaxis (Dreger *et al.* 2003). The cumulative treatment-related mortality was 18% (CI 9–27) with event-free and overall survival at 24 months estimated to be 56% (CI 43–69) and 72% (CI 61–83), respectively. At the moment there is lack of clarity about the optimum conditioning schedule for 'mini' transplant procedures and what approach should be used for GVHD control. A recent unpublished study of the EBMT database comparing low-intensity allogeneic transplantation with standard allografts has suggested that outcomes may be superior using a reduced-intensity protocol (P. Dreger, personal communication). Low-intensity transplants in CLL may be considered in patients who are not able to tolerate 'standard' conditioning regimens. The indications for non-myeloablative transplant are the same as for standard allografting. It is not possible to recommend a particular conditioning regimen and patients should be entered into an appropriate clinical research protocol.

Transplants from unrelated donors

There is very little information on allogeneic transplants from non-human leukocyte antigen (HLA) identical sibling donors in CLL. Small numbers have been reported from the IBMTR (Horowitz *et al.* 2000) and fifteen patients have been reported from Germany (Schetelig *et al.* 2000). Again, follow-up is short but it appears that for some younger patients with high-risk disease unrelated donor transplant may offer the chance of an improved outlook. In a UK study of Campath 1H-, melphalan- and fludarabine-treated non-myeloablative transplants mainly for lymphoma, the HLA-matched unrelated donor transplants fared as well as those from HLA identical sibling donors (Chakraverty *et al.* 2001). It is therefore recommended that unrelated donor allograft is not generally advocated in CLL, but for some younger patients where an autograft is not an option or has failed, a transplant from an unrelated donor may be worthwhile. This should be undertaken only as part of a clinical trial protocol.

References

Barlogie, B., Alexanian, R., Dicke, K. *et al.* (1987). High-dose chemotherapy and autologous marrow transplantation for resistant multiple myeloma. *Blood*, 869–872.

Chakraverty, R., Peggs, K., Chopra, R., Milligan, D., Kottaridis, P. *et al.* (2002). Limiting transplant related mortality following unrelated donor transplantation by using a nonmyeloablative conditioning regimen. *Blood* **99**, 1071–1078.

Cull, G. M., Haynes, A. P., Byrne, J. L., Carter, G. I. Miflin, G., Rebello, P., Hale, G., Waldmann, H. & Russell, N. H. (2000). Preliminary experience of allogeneic stem cell transplantation for lymphoproliferative disorders using BEAM-CAMPATH conditioning: an effective regimen with low procedure-related toxicity. *British Journal of Haematology* **108**, 754–760.

Dreger, P., Brand, R., Hansz, J., Milligan, D., Corradini, P., Finke, J., Deliliers, G. *et al.* (2003). Treatment related mortality and graft versus leukemia effect after allogeneic stem cell transplantation for chronic lymphocytic leukemia using intensity reduced conditioning. *Leukemia* **17**, 841–848.

Dreger, P., Stilgenbauer, S., Benner, A., Ritgen, M., Schmitz, N. & Dohner, H. (2002). High-dose therapy with autologous stem cell transplantation (ASCT) prolongs survival of patients with chronic lymphocytic leukemia (CLL): a matched-pair analysis. *Blood* **100**, 217a (abstract).

Dreger, P. Michallet, M. & Schmitz, N. (2000). Stem-cell transplantation for chronic lymphocytic leukemia: the 1999 perspective. *Annals of Oncology* **11** (Suppl. 1), 49–53.

Dreger, P., van Biezen, A., Brand, R., Esteve, J., Gratwohl, A., Kimby, E., Michallet, M., Milligan, D. (2000). Prognostic factors for survival after autologous stem cell transplantation for chronic lymphocytic leukaemia: the EBMT experience. *Blood* **96** (Suppl. 1), (abstract 2071).

Dreger, P. & Schmitz, N. (1997). The role of stem cell transplantation in the treatment of chronic lymphocytic leukaemia. *Leukemia* **11** (Suppl. 2), S42–S45.

Dreger, P. & Montserrat, E. (2002). Autologous and allogeneic stem cell transplantation for chronic lymphocytic leukemia. *Leukemia* **16**, 985–992.

Dreger, P., von Neuhoff, N., Kuse, R. *et al.* (1998). Early stem cell transplantation for chronic lymphocytic leukaemia: a chance for cure? *British Journal of Cancer* **77**, 2291–2297.

Esteve, J., Villamor, N., Colomer, D., Cervantes, F., Campo, E., Carreras, E. & Montserrat, E. (2001). Stem cell transplantation for chronic lymphocytic leukemia: different outcome after autologous and allogeneic transplantation and correlation with minimal residual disease status. *Leukemia* **15**, 445–451.

Flinn, I. W., Byrd, J. C., Morrison, C., Jamison, J., Diehl, L. F., Murphy, T., Piantadosi, S., Seifter, E., Ambinder, R. F., Vogelsang, G. & Grever, M. R. (2000). Fludarabine and cyclophosphamide with filgrastim support in patients with previously untreated indolent lymphoid malignancies. *Blood* **96**,71–75.

Forsyth, P., Milligan, D., Davies, F. E. *et al.* (2000). High-dose chemo-radiotherapy with autologous stem cell rescue for patients with CLL is an effective and safe means of inducing molecular responses: an MRC pilot study. *Blood* **96** (Suppl. 1), (abstract 3642).

Gale, R. P. & Montserrat, E. (1995). Intensive therapy of chronic lymphocytic leukaemia. *Baillière's Clinical Haematology* **6**, 879–885.

Giralt, S., Thall, P. F., Khouri, I., Wang, X., Braunschweig, I., Ippolitti, C., Claxton, D., Donato, M., Bruton, J., Cohen, A., Davis, M., Andersson, B. S., Anderlini, P., Gajewski, J., Kornblau, S., Andreeff, M., Przepiorka, D., Ueno, N. T., Molldrem, J. & Champlin, R. (2001). Melphalan and purine analog-containing preparative regimens: reduced-intensity conditioning for patients with hematologic malignancies undergoing allogeneic progenitor cell transplantation. *Blood* **97**, 631–637.

Gribben, J. G., Neuberg, D., Soiffer, R. J. *et al.* (1998). Autologous versus allogeneic bone marrow transplantation for patients with poor prognosis chronic lymphocytic leukemia. *Blood* 92 (Suppl. 1), (abstract 1320).

Horowitz, M. M., Montserrat, E., Sobocinski, K., Giralt, S., Khouri, I. F. & Schmitz, N. (2000). Haematopoietic stem cell transplantation for chronic lymphocytic leukemia. *Blood* **96** (Suppl. 1), (abstract 1758).

Ittala, M., Pelliniemi, T., Rajamaki, A. *et al.* (1997). Autologous blood cell transplantation in CLL: response to chemotherapy prior to mobilisation predicts the stem cell yield. *Bone Marrow Transplantation* **19**, 647–651.

Jarque, I., Palau, J., Sanz, G. F., Guinot, M., Gomis, F., Martin, G., Martinez, J. & Sanz, M. A. (1993). Delayed complete response after allogeneic bone marrow transplantation in chronic lymphocytic leukemia. *Blood* **82**, 1036–1038.

Keating M, O'Brien S, Lerner s *et al.* (2000). Combination chemo-antibody therapy with fludarabine, cyclophosphamide and rituximab achieves high CR rate in previously untreated chronic lymphocytic leukemia. *Blood* **96** (Suppl. 1), (abstract 2214).

Kennedy, B., Rawstron, A., Carter, C. *et al.* (2000). Campath-1H with fludarabine: a novel highly active combination in refractory CLL. *Blood* **96**, (Suppl. 1), (abstract 4991).

Ketterer, N., Salles, G., Moullet, I. *et al.* (1998). Factors associated with successful mobilization of peripheral blood progenitor cells in 200 patients with lymphoid malignancies. *British Journal of Haematology* **103**, 235–242.

Khouri, I. F., Keating, M. J., Vriesendorp, H. M., Reading, C. L., Przepiorka, D., Huh, Y. O., Andersson, B. S., van Besien, K. W., Mehra, R. C. & Giralt, S. A. (1994). Autologous and allogeneic bone marrow transplantation for chronic lymphocytic leukemia: preliminary results. *Journal of Clinical Oncology* **12**, 748–758.

Khouri, I. F., Przepiorka, D., van Besien, K., O'Brien, S., Palmer, J. L., Lerner, S., Mehra, R. C., Vriesendorp, H. M., Andersson, B. S., Giralt, S., Korbling, M., Keating, M. J. & Champlin, R. E. (1997). Allogeneic blood or marrow transplantation for chronic lymphocytic leukaemia: timing of transplantation and potential effect of fludarabine on acute graft-versus-host disease. *British Journal of Haematology* **97**, 466–473.

Khouri, I. F., Keating, M. J. & Champlin, R. (1998). Hematopoietic stem cell transplantation for chronic lymphocytic leukemia. *Current Opinion in Haematology* **5**, 454–459.

Kottaridis, P. D., Milligan, D. W., Chopra, R., Chakraverty, R. K., Chakrabarti, S. *et al.* (2000). *In vivo* Campath 1H prevents graft-versus-host disease following non-myeloablative stem cell transplantation. *Blood* **96**, 2419–2425.

Mattsson, J., Uzunel, M., Remberger, M., Ljungman, P., Kimby, E., Ringden, O. & Zetterquist, H. (2000). Minimal residual disease is common after allogeneic stem cell transplantation in patients with B cell chronic lymphocytic leukemia and may be controlled by graft-versus-host disease. *Leukemia* **14**, 247–254.

Mauro, F. R., Foa, R., Giannarelli, D. *et al.* (1999). Clinical characteristics and outcome of young chronic lymphocytic leukemia patients: a single institution study of 204 cases. *Blood* **94**, 448–454.

Mehta, J., Powles, R., Singhal, S., Iveson, T., Treleaven, J. & Catovsky, D. (1996). Clinical and hematologic response of chronic lymphocytic and prolymphocytic leukemia persisting after allogeneic bone marrow transplantation with the onset of acute graft-versus-host disease: possible role of graft-versus-leukemia. *Bone Marrow Transplantation* **17**, 371–375.

Michallet, M., Archimbaud, E., Bandini, G., Rowlings, P. A., Deeg, H. J., Gahrton, G., Montserrat, E., Rozman, C., Gratwohl, A. & Gale, R. P. (1996). HLA-identical sibling bone marrow transplantation in younger patients with chronic lymphocytic leukemia. European Group for Blood and Marrow Transplantation and the International Bone Marrow Transplant Registry.

Michallet, M., van Biezen, A., Bandini, G. *et al.* (1999). Allotransplants and autotransplants in chronic lymphocytic leukaemia (CLL). *Bone Marrow Transplantation* **23**(Suppl. 19), (abstract 795).

Michallet, M., Thiebaud, A., Dreger, P. *et al.* (2000). Peripheral blood stem cell mobilisation and transplantation after fludarabine therapy in chronic lymphocytic leukaemia: A report of the EBMT CLL Subcommittee on behalf of the EBMT Chronic Leukaemia Working Party. *British Journal of Haematology* **108**, 595–601.

Milligan, D. W, Fernandes, S., Dasgupta, R., Davies, F. E., Matutes, E., Fegan, C. D., McConkey, C., Child, J. A., Cunningham, D., Morgan, G. J. & Catovsky, D. (2004). Autografting for younger patients with chronic lymphocytic leukaemia is safe and achieves a high percentage of molecular responses. Results of the MRC Pilot Study. *Blood*. Pre-published online 29.4.04.

Montserrat, E., Esteve, J., Schmitz, N., Dreger, P. *et al.* (1999). Autologous stem cell transplantation in chronic lymphocytic leukaemia; results in 107 patients. *Blood* **94**(Suppl. 1), (abstract 1798).

Pavletic, Z. S., Arrowsmith, E. R., Bierman, P. J., Goodman, S. A., Vose, J. M., Tarantolo, S. R., Stein, R. S., Bociek, G., Greer, J. P., Wu, C. D., Kollath, J. P., Weisenburger, D. D., Kessinger, A., Wolff, S. N., Armitage, J. O. & Bishop, M. R. (2000). Outcome of allogeneic stem cell transplantation for B cell chronic lymphocytic leukemia. *Bone Marrow Transplantation* **25**, 717–722.

Provan, D., Bartlett-Pandite, L., Zwicky, C. *et al.* (1996). Eradication of PCR detectable chronic lymphocytic cells is associated with improved outcome after bone marrow transplantation. *Blood* **88**, 2228–2235.

Rabinowe, S. N., Soiffier, R. J., Gribben, J. *et al.* (1993). Autologous and allogeneic bone marrow transplantation for poor prognosis patients with B-cell chronic leukemia. *Blood* **4**, 1366.

Rai, K. R., Peterson, B. L., Appelbaum, F. R., Kolitz, J., Elias, L., Shepherd, L. *et al.* (2000). Fludarabine compared with chlorambucil therapy for chronic lymphocytic leukemia. *New England Journal of Medicine* **343**, 1750–1757.

Rai, K, Mercia R, Cooper R *et al.* (2000). Campath-1H is an effective salvage therapy for fludarabine failing CLL patients: results of a phase II trial. *Blood* **96**(Suppl. 1), (abstract 705).

Rondon, G., Giralt, S., Huh, Y., Khouri, I., Andersson, B., Andreeff, M., Champlin, R. (1996). Graft-versus-leukemia effect after allogeneic bone marrow transplantation for chronic lymphocytic leukemia. [Case Reports. Journal Article] *Bone Marrow Transplantation* **18**, 669–672.

Rondon, G., Giralt, S., Pereira, M., Van Besien, K., Mehra, R., Champlin, R. & Andreeff, M. (1997). Analysis of chimerism following allogeneic bone marrow transplantation by fluorescent-in-situ hybridization. *Leukemia & Lymphoma* **25**, 463–437.

Ritgen, M., Dreger, P., Humpe, A., Stilgenbauer, S., Döhner, H. & Kneba, M. (2002). Quantitative PCR demonstrates effective graft versus host leukemia activity after allogeneic stem cell transplantation using reduced intensity conditioning in patients with chronic lymphocytic leukemia. *Blood* **100** 854a (abstract).

Ritgen, M., Lange, A., Stilgenbauer, S., Dohner, H., Bretscher, C., Bosse, H., Stuhr, A., Kneba, M. & Dreger, P. (2003). Unmutated immunoglobulin variable heavy-chain gene status remains an adverse prognostic factor after autologous stem cell transplantation for chronic lymphocytic leukemia. *Blood* **101**, 2049–2053.

Sala, R., Mauro, F., Belluci, R. *et al.* (1998). Evaluation of blood and marrow haemopoietic progenitors in chronic lymphocytic leukaemia before and after chemotherapy. *European Journal of Haematology* **61**, 14–20.

Scime, R., Indovina, A., Santoro, A., Musso, M., Olivieri, A., Tringali, S., Crescimanno, A., Montanari, M., Felice, R., Catania, P., Mariani, G., Leoni, P. & Majolino, I. (1998). PBSC mobilization, collection and positive selection in patients with chronic lymphocytic leukemia. *Bone Marrow Transplantation* **22**,1159–1165.

Schetelig, J., Thiede, C., Bornhauser, M., Schwerdtfeger, R., Kiehl, M., Beyer, J., Kroger, N., Hensel, M., Scheffold, C., Ho, A. D., Kienast, J., Neubauer, A., Zander, A. R., Fauser, A. A., Ehninger, G. & Siegert, W. (2002). Reduced non-relapse mortality after reduced intensity conditioning in advanced chronic lymphocytic leukemia. *Annals of Hematology* **81**(Suppl 2), S47–S48.

Stilgenbauer, S., Neuhoff, N., Bullinger, L., Krober, A., Lichter, P., Dreger, P. & Dohner, H. (2000). Deletion 11q23 identifies B-CLL patients at high risk for molecular disease persistance after high dose therapy and autografting. *Blood* **96**, 715a (abstract).

Sutton, L., Maloum, K., Gonzalez, H. *et al.* (1998). Autologous haematopoietic stem cell transplantation as salvage treatment for advanced B cell chronic lymphocytic leukaemia. *Leukemia* **12**, 1699–1707.

van Besien, K., Keralavarma, B., Devine, S. & Stock, W. (2001). Allogeneic and autologous transplantation for chronic lymphocytic leukemia. *Leukemia* **15**, 1317–1325.

Visani, G., Lemoli, R., Tosi, P. *et al.* (1999). Fludarabine containing regimens severely impair peripheral blood stem cell mobilisation and collection in acute myeloid leukemia patients. *British Journal of Haematology* **105**, 775–779.

Chapter 9

Chronic lymphocytic leukaemia: a review of new agents under development

Martin J. S. Dyer

Introduction

The year 2003 marked the 50th anniversary of the discovery of the structure of DNA by Watson and Crick. As it so happens, it also marks the 50th anniversary of the synthesis of the water-soluble aromatic nitrogen mustard derivative *p*-(di-2-chloroethlamino)-phenyl butyric acid (C.B.1348), now known as chlorambucil, a derivative of the group of highly reactive compounds extracted from mustard plants identified by Paul Ehrlich (Figure 9.1 and Everett *et al.* 1953). In initial clinical trials of this agent in chronic lymphocytic leukaemia (CLL), four of the eight patients entered remission (Galton *et al.* 1955). Despite the synthesis of many variants, including antibodies conjugated with chlorambucil, in the UK at least, C.B.1348 remains the standard against which newer pretenders such as fludarabine continue to be compared.

The relative lack of therapeutic progress in CLL over the subsequent 50 years contrasts with that made in childhood acute lymphoblastic leukemia (ALL) (Laszlo 1995) and stems not only from the usual indolent nature of the disease, the chronic immunosuppression and the older age of the CLL patient population, but also from our lack of knowledge concerning the biology of the disease and the nature of the pathways deranged in the pathogenesis of the disease. From cytogenetic analysis, there appears to be no consistent genetic lesion. Moreover, the lesions that have been identified including trisomy of chromosome 12, deletion of chromosome 13q14, 17p13 and 11q23 have either not been amenable to molecular analysis or occur as secondary events, arising in a subpopulation of cells. The recent identification of micro RNAs as the targets of the 13q14 deletions and the recognition of the pivotal roles of such molecules in the control of apoptosis and development may allow new therapeutic approaches (Calin *et al.* 2002; Brennecke *et al.* 2003; Benfey 2003). Generation of transgenic murine models may also be of value; a *TCL1* transgene, expressed in B-cells under the control of the immunoglobulin Eμ enhancer results in the development of a disease that appears to be similar biologically to CLL (Bichi *et al.* 2002).

However, other recent work suggests that CLL may represent a dynamic interplay between tumour and residual normal cells and may therefore not be amenable to such 'simple' genetic analysis. CLL has long been thought of as a disease of altered

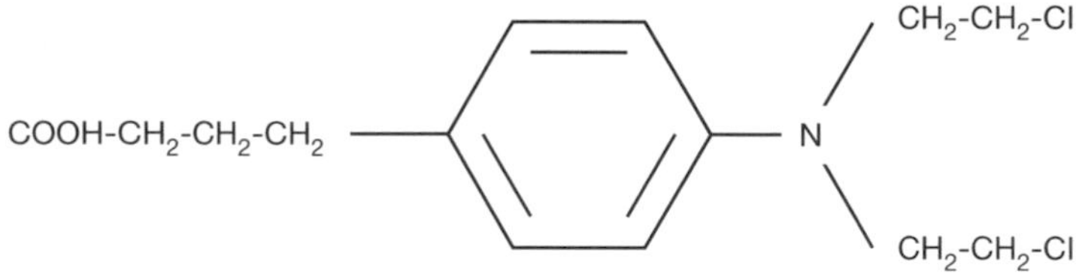

Figure 9.1 Structure of C.B.1348 or chlorambucil.

sensitivity to programmed cell death or apoptosis and the slow accumulation of cells otherwise destined to die (Galton 1966) but this paradigm is being increasingly challenged by several observations. Firstly, preliminary studies using heavy water to label DNA metabolically *in vivo* indicate that the neoplastic clone may turnover in a matter of months (Neese *et al.* 2002; Messmer *et al.* 2002; and www.kinemed.net). Secondly, various data indicate that CLL cells depend for continued survival on interactions with specialised dendritic cells within the peripheral blood, lymph node and bone marrow (Tsukada *et al.* 2002; Burger & Kipps 2002; Woolston *et al.* 2003); such biological complexity would be difficult to model in murine systems. The nature of the crucial interaction(s) remains unclear but candidates include integrin signalling pathways, IL4 and IL7 pathways, as well as the interactions of CXCR4 with SDF1, and TNFSF13B (BLyS) with its various receptors. There is some evidence to suggest that the TNFSF13B cytokine may provide an autocrine 'loop' of importance in the pathogenesis of CLL, comparable to a similar proposed autocrine CD40–CD154 loop in lymphoma (Novak *et al.* 2002; Pham *et al.* 2002). These and other data may provide new therapeutic targets for either small molecule inhibitors or for agonistic/ antagonistic monoclonal antibodies (MAbs) (Bertolini *et al.* 2002). Several companies are now working on means of inhibiting the interactions of the TNFSF13B cytokine for both malignant and non-malignant B-cell conditions (see for example http://www.hgsi.com/products/LSB.html).

A corollary of these observations is that there should be a proliferating CLL stem cell population, which may differ significantly in transcriptome and phenotype from the bulk of cells in the peripheral blood (Reya *et al.* 2001; Decker *et al.* 2003; Albesiano *et al.* 2003). Work from Professor Caligaris-Cappio has shown that cells in lymph node 'proliferation centres' are indeed significantly different having for example increased levels of CD20 expression and lacking p27Kip1 (Ghia and Caligaris-Cappio 2000). Further characterisation of these stem-cell or progenitor populations may suggest additional targets.

On a more practical level, *in vitro* testing of CLL sensitivity to chemotherapeutic agents should be performed in the presence of stromal cell populations since they may significantly alter sensitivity to various drugs; this has been shown in the case of myeloma (Nefedova *et al.* 2003). Work from our own laboratory has shown that culturing CLL in the presence of mesenchymal stem cell populations derived from normal bone marrow protects CLL from the effects of both proteasomal and protein kinase C inhibitors (Woolston *et al.* 2003).

Despite these problems, or perhaps because of them, there are now many compounds under development that may have therapeutic applications in CLL (Table 9.1 and Johnson *et al.* 2003). The purpose of this chapter is to review some, but certainly by no means all, of these new agents and their possible application in CLL. Each class of agent is discussed separately below in no particular order. None of them are specific for the disease and several caveats should be noted. Firstly, many affect many different pathways simultaneously. This appears to be particularly so for the inhibitors of the histone deacetylases, which can influence an almost limitless number of different proteins both inside and outside the nucleus. Moreover, these effects may be cell-type specific, making extrapolation from one set of experiments to another very hazardous. Thirdly, where these compounds have been assessed on primary material from patients with CLL, CLL cells have invariably been cultured without supporting stromal cells, under conditions that may selectively activate certain pathways, which may not necessarily be activated *in vivo* and at low concentrations (usually 10^6 CLL cells/ml) that again do not reflect those seen *in vivo* (Pettitt *et al.* 2001). Fourthly, no account is made in most of these 'pharmacological' studies of the different subtypes of CLL and the possible influences that different genetic differences might make. Finally, 'apoptotic' endpoints used vary and need to be carefully assessed. It is perhaps not surprising then that the results of *in vitro* testing may not necessarily reflect those obtained *in vivo*!

Despite these problems in interpreting the *in vitro* data, many of these agents have entered phase I/II clinical trials. Even if these compounds show little activity by themselves, the hope is that they may enhance the efficacy of regular chemotherapeutic agents without additional toxicities. Numerous studies combining fludarabine or fludarabine/cyclophosphamide regimens with any one of these agents should therefore be anticipated. However, given their multiple sites of action and lack of specificity for CLL, it is difficult to foresee a rational rather than empirical plan of development.

(a) Proteasomal inhibition

Proteasomal inhibition is not an obvious target for therapy of either malignant or non-malignant disorders, but nonetheless has become the centre of much interest recently (Adams 2002; Almond & Cohen 2002). Proteasomes are huge 26S multi-subunit protein complexes where proteins tagged for destruction by specific post-translational modifications are unfolded and degraded. The active site of the proteasomal protease contains a threonine residue that can be specifically inhibited. Inhibition of protein degradation naturally has a huge number of effects within the cell but in terms of cancer therapy, key results are thought to include up-regulation of p53 and the cell

Table 9.1 Some agents in development for treatment of CLL

Agent	Presumed mode of action	Company
Velcade/PS-341	Proteasomal inhibition (?Inhibition of NF-κB pathways)	Millennium www.mlnm.com/
UCN-01 7-hydoxystaurosporine PKC412	CDK inhibitor Protein kinase C inhibitor CHK1 inhibitor	
Synthetic triterpenoids CDDO CDDO-me +/− TRAIL or TRAIL agonistic antibodies	Activation of the extrinsic apoptotic pathway Activation of caspase 8? Down-regulation of cFLIP?	NCI www.hgs.com
17-Aminogeldanamycin	Inhibition of heat shock proteins, especially HSP90	
Depsipeptide NVP-LAQ824 (Valproate!), etc	Histone deacetylase inhibition	Fujisawa NCI Novartis, etc.
G3139 *BCL2* antisense	Down-regulation of anti-apoptotic BCL2 protein	Genta www.genta.com
EB1089 Vitamin D3 analogue		Leo Pharmaceuticals

cycle inhibitor, p27Kip1, while prevention of IκB proteasomal degradation is thought to be essential to abrogate NF-κB activation through retention of the NF-κB transcription factors within the cytoplasm where they cannot mediate their anti-apoptotic effects. Since constitutive NF-κB activation is thought to be an essential pathogenic component of many malignancies of mature B-cells including CLL, suppression of this pathway might provide effective therapy. However, proteasomal inhibition is also toxic to normal cells.

Bortezomib (PS-341; Velcade, Millenium Pharmaceuticals; Figure 9.2) has a high affinity and specificity for the catalytic site of the 26S proteasome. This drug has been trialled in many malignancies but has recently been approved by the US Food and Drug Administration (FDA) in refractory myeloma, where studies show an overall 35% response rate with an apparent 10% complete remission rate as adjudged by absence of paraprotein. Preliminary results in CLL seem to be less promising (Orlowski *et al.* 2002). In this phase I study in various relapsed haematological malignancies, the maximum tolerated dose was 1.04 mg/m^2 given twice weekly for four weeks. Dose-limiting toxicities included thrombocytopaenia and neutropaenia as

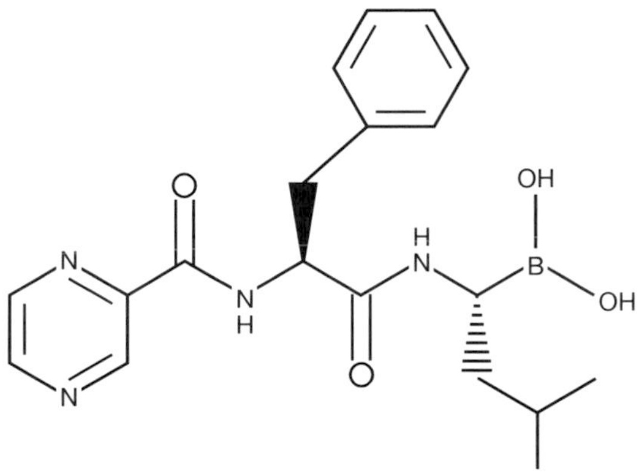

Figure 9.2 Structure of the proteasomal inhibitor PS-341.

well as peripheral neuropathy, hyponatraemia, hypokalaemia, fatigue, and malaise. Although these data would seem to preclude a use for this drug on its own for CLL, it may be useful in enhancing sensitivity to other apoptosis-inducing agents, perhaps using lower and less toxic schedules. As an example of this kind of sensitisation, CLL cells are normally almost completely resistant to TRAIL-mediated apoptosis (mediated through the extrinsic pathway) despite expressing cell surface receptors (MacFarlane *et al.* 2002). The molecular nature of this resistance is not clear. Co-culture of cells with PS-341 and TRAIL has been reported to enhance sensitivity by reducing levels of the apoptotic inhibitory protein, cFLIP (Sayers *et al.* 2003); however, it is not apparent how this might occur because cFLIP is thought to undergo proteasomal degradation, and consequently, levels might be anticipated to rise with PS-341.

(b) PI-3 kinase and protein kinase C inhibition

There are several lines of evidence to suggest that PI-3 kinase and Protein kinase C might be interesting targets for the treatment of CLL. PI-3 kinase appears to be consitutively active in CLL, although the mechanisms underlying this activation are not yet clear. Activation of PI-3 kinase appears to result in activation of some isoforms of protein kinase C delta, but interestingly (given the high levels of TCL1 expression in CLL B-cells) not AKT, which remains minimally phosphorylated. Suppression of PI-3 kinase or PKC delta *in vitro* result in apoptosis of CLL cells (Ringshausen *et al.* 2002). Moreover, several groups have shown that inhibition of PKC delta sensitises cells to the cytotoxic effects of fludarabine *in vitro* (Barragan *et al.* 2002). Clinical effects of PKC inhibition with the inhibitor PKC412 in a phase I study were quite modest (Virchis *et al.* 2002). Interestingly, a recent preliminary *in vitro* study has suggested a possible synergistic interaction between UCN-01 (or 7-hydroxystaurosporine) and the heat shock protein 90 (HSP90) antagonist, 17-allyl-aminogeldanamycin (17-AAG) (Jia *et al.* 2003). Synergy appeared to occur independently of protein kinase C inhibition. Inhibition of HSP90 by geldanamycin and its derivatives is a novel target in its own right (Blagosklonny 2002). These yeast-derived antibiotic compounds target the 'molecular chaperones' including HSP90 and the related GRP9 and its homologues. These proteins are involved in correct molecular folding and therefore function, of interacting proteins including p53 and other important modulators of cell division and apoptosis; inactivation of the HSP90 chaperone results in rapid degradation, usually via the proteasome, and may thus lead to cell death. Clincal studies of 17-AAG have been initiated in the USA and in the UK although not in CLL so far.

(c) Synthetic triterpenoids (CDDO)

Triterpenoids are a class of naturally occurring compounds that have anti-tumour activity. Synthetic variants including 2-cyano-3, 12-dioxoolean-1,9-dien-28-oic acid (CDDO) and its methyl ester derivative (CDDO-me), generated in the laboratory of Dr Sporn, have recently been tested *in vitro* for their ability to induce apoptosis of a variety of leukaemic cells. Both CDDO and CDDO-me appear to be active against some CLL cells and apparently induce apoptosis through activation of caspase 8 and down-regulation of c-FLIP without obvious activation of caspase 9 (Pedersen *et al.* 2002) i.e. by activation of the extrinsic pathway of apoptosis rather than the more usual mitochondrial, intrinsic pathway. How this might be achieved is not yet clear. However, these data suggest that additional stimulation of the extrinsic pathway, for instance through cell surface receptors such as TRAIL, might synergise with CDDO; preliminary data in acute myeloid leukemia (AML) and in some cases of CLL would appear to support this contention (Pedersen *et al.* 2002; Kim *et al.* 2002; Suh *et al.* 2003). Clinical trials of these agents in haematological malignancies are now starting at the National Cancer Institute (NCI).

(d) Histone deacetylase inhibition

There is currently intense interest in the use of histone deacetylase (HDAC) inhibitors in the treatment of various haematological malignancies and in particular the acute leukaemias, where transcriptional repression appears to be a mechanism common to several oncogenic leukaemia-specific fusion transcripts (Melnick & Licht 2002). The fusion proteins recruit HDACs to specific target genes, repress transcription and suppress normal differentiation. HDACs remove acetyl groups from conserved lysine residues in histones and also in transcription factors including p53 and BCL6. Inhibition of histone deacetylation may not only relieve the differentiation block but may also directly induce apoptosis.

Given that there are three distinct HDAC protein families each with several family members, each present in several different protein isoforms, it is not surprising that there are several different classes of HDAC inhibitors (HDIs) with very diverse chemical structures (Marks *et al.* 2000; Melnick & Licht 2002). The structures of some of these are shown in Figure 9.3. It is of some considerable interest that the eight-carbon branched chain fatty acid sodium valproate or 2-propylpentanoic acid, (which is commonly used in the treatment of some forms of epilepsy and incidentally was first synthesised in 1882!) has recently been shown to be an HDI with the ability in combination with retinoids to cause both derived acute leukaemic cell lines and fresh leukaemic blasts to undergo differentiation *in vitro* at concentrations used to treat epilepsy (Gottlicher *et al.* 2001). Thus, sodium valproate may be an 'off-the-shelf' HDI and is currently in phase I/II trials in combination with ATRA in AML in the USA. Its potential role in CLL has yet to be assessed. It should be noted however that relatively high (micromolar) concentrations are necessary to induce apoptosis *in vitro*.

On the other hand, another HDI, depsipeptide (FR901228), originally isolated from *Chromobacterium violaceum*, is now in phase I clinical trials not only in CLL but also in several other haematological malignancies and appears to be effective at nanomolar concentrations (Nakajima *et al.* 1998). Initial *in vitro* work (Byrd *et al.* 1999) showed an LD_{50} of approximately 40 nM against CLL cells, whereas against normal lymphocytes and bone marrow progenitor populations the LD_{50} was about 100-fold greater. Subsequently, the same group have shown that the concentrations used resulted in histone H3 and H4 acetylation and HDAC inhibition, as anticipated, but in addition, activated apoptosis through the extrinsic pathway by caspase 8 and caspase 3; these data were unanticipated. In their hands, depsipeptide resulted in early down-regulation of the anti-apoptotic cFLIP protein, before overt apoptosis was induced, without any corresponding changes of either CD95 (Fas) receptor expression or in any other apoptotic proteins including BCL2, BAX, MCL1 and XIAP (Aron *et al.* 2003). These data might indicate a potential synergy with tumour necrosis factor (TNF)-α-mediated apoptosis induction. Trials of this interesting agent are now ongoing in CLL (Bruner *et al.* 2002). One patient with chemotherapy-resistant peripheral T-cell lymphoma attained a complete response with depsipeptide (Piekarz *et al.* 2001).

As noted above, much remains to be discovered about the mode(s) of action of the HDIs. Given their very different structures and probable different specificities, lessons learnt from one HDI in a particular clinical situation may not apply to another. There is now debate over whether transcription is the primary target for HDIs (Johnstone & Licht 2003). HDIs may influence transcription and reverse repression in some instances but it also seems likely that they may induce p21 to cause G1 arrest and differentiation and may also cause pro-apoptotic genes and proteins to be induced as well. Moreover, recent work in CML indicates that one HDI, LAQ824 (Novartis) can both lower expression and promote proteasomal degradation (through acetylation of the chaperone protein hsp90) of the BCR-ABL fusion protein in cultured and primary blast-crisis cells (Nimmanapalli *et al.* 2003). Similarly, in lung cancer cells,

Name	Structure

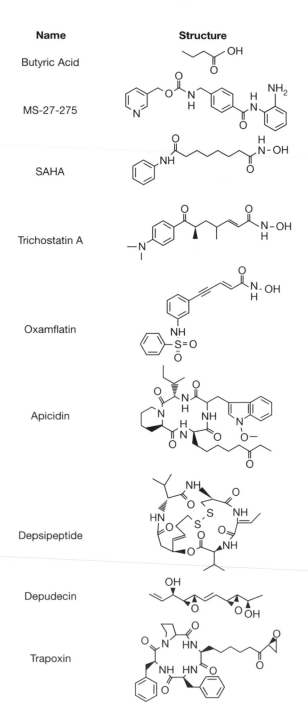

Butyric Acid

MS-27-275

SAHA

Trichostatin A

Oxamflatin

Apicidin

Depsipeptide

Depudecin

Trapoxin

Figure 9.3 Structures of some histone deacetylase inhibitors.

depsipeptide acetylated the hsp90 protein, resulting in destabilisation of several proteins resulting in their proteasomal degradation; these proteins included mutant p53 as well as ERBB1 and B2 and RAF1 (Yu *et al.* 2002). Finally, there is the prospect of synergistic interactions between HDIs and DNA demethylating agents. Apart from hypoacetylation, transcriptional repression of key target genes such as *CDKN2* may be mediated by hypermethylation. Expression of such hypoacetylated and hypermethylated genes may be best achieved by using a combination of HDIs and 5-Azacytidine, which sequesters DNA methyltransferases (Jones & Baylin 2002).

(e) Antisense inhibition of anti-apoptotic protein expression

BCL2 is a 26 kDa protein associated with the outer mitochondrial membrane that protects a variety of cell types from apoptosis. BCL2 defines a family of structurally-related proteins, which can be either anti- or pro-apoptotic. BCL2 over-expression occurs in B-cell lymphomas as a consequence of the chromosomal translocation t(14;18)(q32;q21) and in CLL through promoter hypomethylation; very high levels of BCL2 are seen in CLL. Down-regulation of BCL2 might therefore result directly in apoptosis or to increased sensitivity to other apoptotic agents.

Oblimersen sodium (G3139; Genasense, Genta Pharmaceuticals, www.genta.com/) is a *BCL2* antisense oligonucleotide (ASO) that has been widely used both *in vitro* and *in vivo* (Waters *et al.* 2000). The high level expression of BCL2 in most cases of CLL makes this a particularly good disease for studying efficacy and a Phase III study assessing the value of G3139 in combination with fludarabine and cyclophosphamide in relapsed patients has recently been completed. Results should be available at ASH later this year. Similar trials have been conducted in myeloma and in melanoma. Provisional results from the latter comparing the addition of G3139 to dacarbazine-based chemotherapy for advanced melanoma showed a slight prolongation in survival (http://www.genta.com/Genta/InvestorRelation/2003/press_20030910_1.html).

Other potential targets for an antisense approach would be MCL1, another BCL2 anti-apoptotic family member; the short half-life of the MCL1 protein and the association of MCL1 down-regulation with apoptosis induction might make it a particularly good target for this approach.

However, it is not clear that such ASOs act by specifically down-regulating the target gene; if this were the case one would anticipate a much more severe toxicity profile, because BCL2 is widely expressed. Another possibility altogether is that ASOs may act as CpG oligonucleotides to stimulate innate immune mechanisms through the Toll receptors. Unmethylated CpG dinucelotides derived from bacteria and synthetic oligonucleotides are able to activate immune effector cells and enhance anti-tumour cytotoxicity, the effects varying according to the sequence of the DNA. Two different types of response have been noted: CpG A oligos inducing IFN-α production and NK activity, whereas type B induce B-cell activation and Th1 cytokines. CpG oligonucleotides may have efficacy on their own but are now being trialled in combination with antibody therapy and chemotherapy of lymphomas (Jahrsdorfer & Weiner 2003).

(f) Vitamin D3 analogues

Vitamin D3 receptors are expressed on a variety of normal and malignant cells, and exposure to 1,25 $(OH)_2$ D3 can inhibit proliferation, induce differentiation and apoptosis in several cell types. Analogues of this compound have been synthesised that exhibit enhanced anti-tumour activity and diminished or absent hypercalcaemic activity. The relatively high levels of VDR expression in CLL cells compared with normal B-cells and T-cells prompted the investigation of one such analogue, EB1089 *in vitro* (Pepper *et al.* 2003). EB1089 was able to induce apoptosis in all 102 CLL samples tested at low concentration (LD_{50} of approximately 20 nM); under the same conditions, normal lymphocytes exhibited an LD_{50} of about 40 nM. EB1089 induced apoptosis in a caspase-dependent but apparently p53-independent fashion, through phosphorylation of p38 MAPK leading to downstream inhibition of ERK. Clinical studies with this agent and other derivatives are awaited.

(g) Monoclonal antibodies

Anti-tumour MAbs may function either through activation of natural effector mechanisms such as antibody-dependent cellular cytotoxicity (ADCC) and complement-mediated lysis or through induction of apoptosis. There are currently no MAbs specific for CLL B-cells, although many different MAbs are now being assessed in clinical trials in the USA. Proteomic analysis of the CLL cell surface membrane has recently identified several new molecules that may be targeted therapeutically (Boyd *et al.* 2003).

Of the currently available MAbs, the CD52 MAb CAMPATH-1H has significant efficacy against haematological disease, even in patients with p53 mutations and in younger patients, can be used to consolidate partial remissions prior to high-dose therapy. In some patients, the level of remission attained within the bone marrow appears to be below the level of 1 malignant cell per 10^4 or 10^5 normal cells. Nevertheless, such patients still relapse, presumably from MAb 'sanctuary' sites. Whether radiolabelled CAMPATH-1 MAbs would be effective consolidation therapy in this setting is not known. The more widespread use of CAMPATH-1H is compromised by its lack of efficacy against lymph nodal disease and by the resulting profound immunosuppression. The CD20 chimaeric MAb rituximab shows little activity against CLL (Mavromatis & Cheson 2003), whilst preliminary data indicate that the CD22 MAb epratuzamab, may have a similar lack of activity in this disease (Leonard *et al.* 2003). IDEC-152 is a novel 'primatised' CD23 MAb that has been shown to induce apoptosis of CLL cells *in vitro*; this MAb is now being assessed in clinical trials (Hopkins *et al.* 2002). Whereas the CD23 molecule is expressed at high levels in CLL, levels of CD23 in the circulation may impede clinical activity. MAbs against the invariant component of HLADR may not be most obvious therapeutic target, because this molecule is expressed on range of normal tissues, including renal endothelium. Nevertheless, HLADR MAbs may be of clinical interest as they induce apoptosis by a mitochondrial but caspase-independent mechanism and may thus synergise with other agents (Bains *et al.* 2003). 'Second generation' MAbs are now being generated with either enhanced affinity (http://www.genmab.com/view_news. asp?filID=121) or with improved Fc-binding through correct glycosylation (http://www.glycart.com/). *In vitro* they would appear to eliminate CLL cells under conditions when their parental constructs are inactive; whether these constructs will be markedly superior *in vivo* remains to be determined.

Both CD20 and CD52 MAbs are now being tested in combination with fludarabine-based regimens. *In vitro*, some CLL cells show evidence of down-regulation of antiapoptotic proteins MCL1 and XIAP as well as activation of caspases 3 and 9 after exposure to rituximab (Byrd *et al.* 2002); this may provide a biological basis for the use of this MAb in combination with fludarabine and cyclophosphamide. Similarly, CAMPATH-1H may synergise with fludarabine; this combination will be tested in the UK (Kennedy *et al.* 2002; and http://www.ukcll.org/ camflud.html).

Future prospects: a personal perspective

The development of curative treatment strategies for ALL proceeded along empirical lines (Laszlo 1995). In the post-genomic era this approach is no longer acceptable. The elderly and chronically immunocompromised patient with CLL presents specific problems. It is likely that to cure CLL will require tumour-targeted therapy but this still appears remote. The trend in chemotherapy just now is to use purine-based combinations with or without MAbs. Although this may improve rates of remission induction, there is currently no evidence that this approach prolongs survival and it may have deleterious effects on normal haemopoietic reserves. The paradigm we should now be following is that of the development of specific kinase inhibitors for CML based on the structure of the BCR-ABL tyrosine kinase, but a similarly amenable and specific target for CLL appears to be lacking.

None of the approaches mentioned above represent tumour-specific therapy, and it seems unlikely that any one alone will be curative. The HDAC inhibitors are of most interest because they appear to be able to influence so many pathways concurrently.

The era of combination therapy for CLL is now upon us, at least for younger patients, but selecting prospectively the correct combinations for a specific subtype of disease should demand prior *in vitro* testing under defined conditions.

Attempts to generate anti-CLL immunity using virally infected cells are cumbersome and, thus far, limited in efficacy (Kipps *et al.* 2000). Nevertheless, the Achilles' heel of CLL appears to be the induction of apoptosis. Concurrent activation of multiple pro-apoptotic molecules and pathways either by small molecules or by antibodies to cell-surface signal transduction molecules, or perhaps by using intracellular targeting with single-chain antibody constructs (Lobato & Rabbitts 2003), should be possible. Alternatively, targeting of the B-cell receptor for antigen may also be effective (Chiorazzi and Ferrarini 2003) at delivering genuinely targeted therapy.

Final word

If the prospects are confusing for the physicians, the situation can only be worse for the patients! A patient-led website (www.clltopics.org) is highly recommended; 'Project Alpha', which is currently under discussion, is an interesting patient-led and sponsored therapeutic proposal.

Acknowledgements

The author gratefully acknowledges the support and encouragement of Professor Gerry Cohen and colleagues at the MRC Toxicology Unit, Leicester, and the financial support from the Medical Research Council, the Leukaemia Research Fund, and the Association for International Cancer Research.

References

Adams, J. (2002). Proteasome inhibitors as new anticancer drugs. *Current Opinions in Oncology* **14**, 628–634.

Albesiano, E. *et al.* (2003). Activation induced cytidine deaminase in chronic lymphocytic leukemia B cells: expression as multiple forms in a dynamic, variably sized fraction of the clone. *Blood* **102**, 3333–3339.

Almond, J. B. & Cohen, G. M. (2002). The proteasome: a novel target for cancer chemotherapy. *Leukemia* **16**, 433–443.

Aron J. L. *et al.* (2003). Depsipeptide (FR901288) induces histone acetylation and inhibition of histone deacetylase in chronic lymphocytic leukemia cells concurrent with activation of caspase 8-mediated apoptosis and down-regulation of cFLIP protein. *Blood* **102**, 652–658.

Bains S. K. *et al.* (2003). Mitochondria control of cell death induced by anti-HLA-DR antibodies. *Leukemia* **17**, 1357–1365.

Barragan M. *et al.* (2002). Involvement of protein kinase C and phosphatidylinositol 3-kinase pathways in the survival of B-cell chronic lymphocytic leukemia cells. *Blood* **99**, 2969–2976.

Benfey, P. N. (2003). MicroRNA is here to stay. *Nature* **425**, 244–245.

Bertolini, F. *et al.* (2002). CXCR4 neutralization, a novel therapeutic approach for non-Hodgkin's lymphoma. *Cancer Research* **62**, 3106–3112.

Bichi, R. *et al.* (2002). Human chronic lymphocytic leukemia modeled in mouse by targeted *TCL1* expression. *Proceedings of the National Academy of Sciences of the United States of America* **99**, 6955–6960.

Blagosklonny, M. V. (2002). HSP-90 associated oncoproteins: multiple targets of geldanamycin and its analogs. *Leukemia* **16**, 455–462.

Boyd, R. S. *et al.* (2003). Proteomic analysis of the cell-surface membrane in chronic lymphocytic leukemia: identification of two novel proteins, BCNP1 and MIG2B. *Leukemia* **17**, 1605–1612.

Brennecke, J. *et al.* (2003). Bantam encodes a developmentally regulated microRNA that controls cell proliferation and regulates the proapoptotic gene hid in *Drosophila*. *Cell* **113**, 25–36.

Bruner, R. J. *et al.* (2002). Phase I trial of the histone deacetylase inhibitor depsipeptide (FR901228) in fludarabine-refractory chronic lymphocytic leukemia. *Blood* **100** (Suppl. 1), 385a (abstract).

Burger, J. A. & Kipps, T. J. (2002). Chemokine receptors and stromal cells in the homing and homeostasis of chronic lymphocytic leukemia B cells. *Leukemia and Lymphoma* **43**, 461–466.

Byrd, J. C. *et al.* (1999). Depsipeptide (FR901228): a novel therapeutic agent with selective in vitro activity against human B-cell chronic lymphocytic leukaemia cells. *Blood* **94**, 1401–1408.

Byrd, J. C. *et al.* (2002). The mechanism of tumor cell clearance by rituximab *in vivo* in patients with chronic lymphocytic leukemia: evidence for caspase activation and apoptosis induction. *Blood* **99**, 1038–1043.

Calin, G. A. *et al.* (2002). Frequent deletions and down-regulation of micro-RNA genes miR15 and miR16 at 13q14 in chronic lymphocytic leukemia. *Proceedings of the National Academy of Sciences of the United States of America* **99**, 15,524–15,529.

Chiorazzi, N. & Ferrarini, M. (2003). B-cell chronic lymphocytic leukemia: lessons learned from the study of the B-cell antigen receptor. *Annual Review of Immunology* **21**, 841–894.

Decker T. *et al.* (2003). Rapamycin-induced G1 arrest in cycling B-CLL cells is associated with reduced expression of Cyclin D3, cyclin E, cyclin A and surviving. *Blood* **101**, 278–285.

Everett, J. L., Roberts, J. J. & Ross, W. C. J. (1953). Aryl-2-halogenalkylamines. Part XII. Some carboxylic derivatives of NN-di-2-chloroethylaniline. *Journal of the Chemical Society* 2386.

Galton, D. A. G. *et al.* (1955). Clinical trials of *p*-(di-2-chloroethlamino)-phenyl butyric acid (C.B.1348) in malignant lymphoma. *British Medical Journal* **2**, 1172–1176.

Galton, D. A. G. (1966) The pathogenesis of chronic lymphocytic leukaemia. *Canadian Medical Association Journal* **94**, 1005–1010.

Ghia, P. & Caligaris-Cappio, F. (2000). The indispensable role of microenvironment in the natural history of low-grade B-cell neoplasms. *Advances in Cancer Research* **79**, 157–173.

Gottlicher, M. *et al.* (2001). Valproic acid defines a novel class of HDAC inhibitors inducing differentiation of transformed cells. *EMBO Journal* **20**, 6969–6978.

Hopkins, M. T. *et al.* (2002). IDEC-152 (anti-CD23) triggers apoptosis of chronic lymphocytic leukaemia cells in vitro. *Blood* **100** (Suppl. 1) 597a (abstract).

Jahrsdorfer, B. & Weiner G. J. (2003). Immunostimulatory CpG oligodeoxynucleotides and antibody therapy of cancer. *Seminars in Oncology* **30**, 476–482.

Jia, W. *et al.* (2003). Synergistic antileukemic interactions between 17-AAG and UCN-01 involve interruption of RAF/MEK and AKT-related pathways. *Blood* **102**, 1824–1832.

Johnson, A. J. *et al.* (2003). Advances in the therapy of chronic lymphocytic leukaemia. *Current Opinions in Hematology* **10**, 297–305.

Johnstone, R. W & Licht J. D. (2003). Histone deacetylase inhibitors in cancer therapy: is transcription the primary target? *Cancer Cell* **4**, 13–18.

Jones, P. A. & Baylin, S. B. (2002). The fundamental role of epigenetic events in cancer. *Nature Reviews Genetics* **3**, 415–428.

Kennedy, B. *et al.* (2002). CAMPATH-1H and fludarabine in combination are highly active in refractory chronic lymphocytic leukaemia. *Blood* **99**, 2245–2247.

Kim, Y. *et al.* (2002). An inducible pathway for degradation of FLIP protein sensitizes tumor cells to TRAIL-induced apoptosis. *Journal of Biological Chemistry* **277**, 22,320–22,329.

Kipps, T. J. *et al.* (2000). Immunogenetic therapy for B-cell malignancies. *Seminars in Oncology* **27** (Suppl. 12), 104–109.

Laszlo, J. (1995). The cure of childhood leukaemia – into the age of miracles. New Brunswick, New Jersey: Rutgers University Press.

Leonard, J. P. *et al*: (2003). Phase I and II trial of epratuzumab (humanized anti-CD22 antibody) in indolent non-Hodgkin's lymphoma. *Journal of Clinical Oncology* **21**, 3051–3059.

Lobato, M. N. & Rabbitts, T. H. (2003). Intracellular antibodies and challenges facing their use as therapeutic agents. *Trends in Molecular Medicine* **9**, 390–396.

MacFarlane, M. *et al.* (2002). Mechanisms of resistance to TRAIL-induced apoptosis in primary B cell chronic lymphocytic leukaemia. *Oncogene* **21**, 6809–6818.

Marks, P. A. *et al.* (2000). Histone Deacetylase Inhibitors: inducers of differentiation or apoptosis of transformed cells. *Journal of the National Cancer Institute* **92**, 1210–1216.

Mavromatis, B. & Cheson, B. D. (2003). Monoclonal antibody therapy of chronic lymphocytic leukemia. *Journal of Clinical Oncology* **21**, 1874–1881.

Melnick, A. & Licht, J. D. (2002). Histone deacetylases as therapeutic targets in haematological malignancies. *Current Opinions in Hematology* **9**, 322–332.

Messmer, D. *et al.* (2002). Direct measurement of B-CLL cell production and turnover *in vivo*. *Blood* **100** (Suppl. 1), 634a (abstract).

Nakajima, H. *et al.* (1998). FR901228, a potent anti-tumor antibiotic, is a novel histone deacetylase inhibitor. *Experimental Cell Research* **241**, 126–133.

Neese, R. A. *et al.* (2002). Measurement *in vivo* of proliferation rates of slow turnover cells by $2H_2O$ labeling of the deoxyribose moiety of DNA. *Proceedings of the National Academy of Sciences of the United States of America* **99**, 15,345–15,350.

Nefedova, Y. *et al.* (2003). Bone marrow stromal-derived soluble factors and direct cell contact contribute to *de novo* drug resistance of myeloma cells by distinct mechanisms. *Leukemia* **17**, 1175–1182.

Nimmanapalli, R. *et al.* (2003). Histone deacetylase inhibitor LAQ824 both lowers expression and promotes protesomal degradation of BCR-ABL and induces apoptosis of imatinib mesylate-sensitive or refractory chronic myelogenous leukemia-blast crisis cells. *Cancer Research* **63**, 5126–5135.

Novak, A. J. *et al.* (2002). Aberrant expression of B-lymphocyte stimulator by B chronic lymphocytic leukemia cells: a mechanism for survival. *Blood* **100**, 2973–2979.

Orlowski, R. Z. *et al.* (2002). Phase I trial of the proteasomal inhibitor PS-341 in patients with refractory haematological malignancies. *Journal of Clinical Oncology* **20**, 4420–4427.

Pedersen, I. M. *et al.* (2002). The triterpenoid CDDO induces apoptosis in refractory CLL B-cells. *Blood* **100**, 2965–2972.

Pepper, C. *et al.* (2003). The vitamin D3 analog EB1089 induces apoptosis via a p53-independent mechanism involving p38 MAP kinase activation and suppression of ERK activity in B-cell chronic lymphocytic leukemia cells *in vitro*. *Blood* **101**, 2454–2460.

Pettitt A.R., Moran E.C. and Cawley J.C. (2001). Homotypic interactions protect chronic lymphocytic leukaemia cells from spontaneous death in vitro. *Leukemia Research* **25**, 1003–1012.

Pham, L. V. *et al.* (2002). A CD40 Signalosome anchored in lipid rafts leads to constitutive activation of NF-κB and autonomous cell growth in B cell lymphomas. *Immunity* **16**, 37–50.

Piekarz, R. L. *et al.* (2001). Inhibitor of histone deacetylation, depsipeptide (FR901228), in the treatment of peripheral and cutaneous T-cell lymphoma: a case report. *Blood* **98**, 2865–2868.

Reya, T. *et al.* (2001) Stem cells, cancer and cancer stem cells. *Nature* **414**, 105–111.

Ringshausen, I. *et al.* (2002). Constitutively activated phophatidylinositol-3 kinase (PI-3K) is involved in the defect of apoptosis B-CLL: association with protein kinase C delta. *Blood* **100**, 3741–3748.

Sayers, T. J. *et al.* (2003). The proteasome inhibitor PS-341 sensitizes neoplastic cells to TRAIL-mediated apoptosis by reducing levels of c-FLIP. *Blood* **102**, 303–310.

Suh, W.-S. *et al.* (2003). Synthetic triterpenoids activate a pathway for apoptosis in AML cells involving downregulation of FLIP and sensitization to TRAIL. *Leukemia* **17**, 1–8.

Tsukada, N. *et al.* (2002). Distinctive features of "nurselike" cells that differentiate in the context of chronic lymphocytic leukemia. *Blood* **99**, 1030–1037.

Virchis, A. *et al.* (2002). A novel treatment approach for low-grade lymphoproliferative disorders using PKC412 (CGP41251) an inhtibitor of protein kinase C. *Hematology Journal* **3**, 131–136.

Waters, J. S. *et al.* (2000). Phase I clinical and pharmacokinetic study of bcl-2 antisense oligonucleotide therapy in patients with non-Hodgkin's lymphoma. *Journal of Clinical Oncology* **18**, 1812–1823.

Woolston, C. M. *et al.* (2003). Bone marrow mesenchymal cells protect chronic lymphocytic leukaemia (CLL) from spontaneous and drug-induced apoptosis. *British Journal of Haematology* **121** (Suppl. 1), (abstract 261).

Yu, X *et al.* (2002). Modulation of p53, ErbB1, ErbB2 and Raf1 expression in lung cancer cells by depsipeptide FR901228. *Journal of the National Cancer Institute* **94**, 504–513.

Chapter 10

The management of immunodeficiency in patients with B-cell chronic lymphocytic leukaemia

Paul Moss

Introduction

Improvements in the supportive case of patients with haematological malignancy have made a major contribution to the improvements in survival that have been seen over the last few years. However, infection remains a significant cause of morbidity and mortality in patients with B-cell chronic lymphocytic leukaemia (B-CLL). Susceptibility to infection in patients with B-CLL is a result of two major factors. The first is the intrinsic state of immunosuppression that is associated with the B-CLL disease process and the second, and perhaps more important, factor is the damage to the immune system that is mediated by treatment of the disease.

The problem of infection in patients with B-CLL

Any healthcare worker who cares for patients with B-CLL can attest to the increased frequency and severity of infection in this group of patients (Tsiodras *et al.* 2000; Morra *et al.* 1999; Molica *et al.* 1993; Robertson 1990). Such an association was reported as far back as the 1950s but is was not until the work of Twomey and others in 1973 that evidence of an increased incidence of infection compared with an age-matched control group was confirmed (Twomey 1973). The study compared B-CLL patients with a control group who had been admitted to hospital with episodes of myocardial infarction. When the number of infections per year in the two patient groups was compared it was clear that B-CLL was associated with an increased incidence of infection across all age groups (Figure 10.1). However, the incidence was particularly marked in patients aged over 70 years and this has been confirmed in subsequent studies (Morrison *et al.* 2001). It should be noted that this study took place in the age when chlorambucil was the major therapeutic option and with the introduction of increasingly intensive chemotherapy agents into the routine management of B-CLL the problem of infection has become more acute than ever.

Infectious episodes are not seen in all patients but it is difficult to predict those patients in whom this will become an issue. Hypogammaglobulinaemia is a risk factor with low predictive value but measurement of the antibody responses to infectious agents such as pneumococcus may be of help (Griffiths *et al.* 1992).

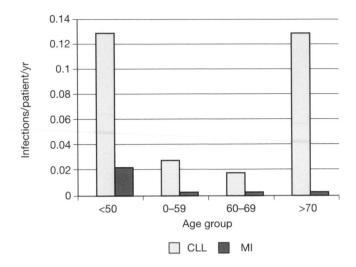

Figure 10.1 Incidence of infection in patients with B-CLL compared with an age-matched control group with myocardial infarction (after Twomey 1973).

The spectrum of infections seen in patients with B-CLL

The most common form of infectious episode seen in patients with B-CLL is bacterial infection of the respiratory tract (Egerer *et al.* 2001; Ahmed *et al.* 2003). In addition, bacterial infection of the skin and urinary tract are relatively frequent events. It is of interest that this pattern of infection is actually very similar to that seen in patients with primary hypogammaglobulinaemia and suggests that humoral deficiency is critical in determining susceptibility to infection.

Although bacterial infection remains a predominant concern throughout the natural history of B-CLL, viral infection is seen much more commonly in patients who have undergone treatment for their disease. Reactivation of herpes viruses is a particular feature. These agents enter a state of latency after infection and the immune system plays an important role in controlling viral replication. Herpes zoster is a common complication of B-CLL and is often associated with disabling and painful symptoms. Reactivation of herpes simplex is observed frequently although drug therapy is usually effective. Over the past few years cytomegalovirus (CMV) has emerged as a significant problem in patients undergoing treatment with lymphocytotoxic antibodies. In addition, its covert role in contributing to disordered immune homeostasis is coming under increasing scrutiny (see below). A wide range of opportunistic infections have also been reported, including *Cryptococcus* (Melzer *et al.* 1998), *Listeria*, *Pneumocystis carinii*, respiratory syncitial virus (RSV) (Eftekhari *et al.* 1998) and tuberculosis (Ghosh *et al.* 1995).

Immunodeficiency in patients with B-CLL

The immune system is essential for the protection of the host from infection and consists of two major arms, the innate and adaptive responses, which are linked at several levels. There is evidence for dysfunction of many arms of the immune system in patients with B-CLL although it is important to separate the influence of treatment from endogenous defects (Chapel & Bunch 1987). In the following section I shall address the innate immune response before coming onto the two major arms of the adaptive immune response, namely the humoral and cellular immune responses.

The innate immune system

Physical barriers to infection are generally well protected in patients with B-CLL although skin lesions and the damaging effect of chemotherapy on highly proliferative cells such as bronchial and gut epithelium may lead to portals for entry of infection. Variations in complement level has been reported in B-CLL and may be potentially relevant to both the disease prognosis (Shvidel et al. 1998) and the efficacy of antibody directed therapies. Functional activation of the complement system as measured by C3b binding to bacteria is also impaired (Heath and Cheson 1985). Natural killer cell function has been reported consistently as defective in B-CLL (Sorskaar et al. 1988; Kimby et al. 1989) and this appears to be largely the result of impaired production or release of cytotoxic mediators after target recognition (Katrinakis et al. 1996). In contrast, neutrophil numbers and function are often preserved in the early phase of disease (Boggs 1960) but decline after disease progression and therapy (Sudhoff et al. 1997). The presence of activated T-cell clones has been associated with the onset of neutropenia (Katrinakis et al. 1995).

Humoral Immunity

B-CLL is characterised by massive expansion of a B-lymphocyte clone but this is associated with significant functional impairment of the residual normal B-cell pool (Jim & Reinhard 1956). Hypogammaglobulinaemia is a frequent and significant complication of B-CLL (Itala et al. 1992) and may involve all of the immunoglobulin isotypes (Lacombe et al. 1999; Copson et al. 1994). The incidence of hypogamma-globulinaemia rises with progression of the disease and reaches approximately 70% after 9 years in untreated patients (Figure 10.2) (Rozman et al. 1988). Hypogammaglobulinaemia is associated with impaired survival and although both IgG and IgA levels have been demonstrated as independent risk factors in one report, only IgA was significant using analysis by multivariate modelling (Rozman et al. 1988). The aetiology of hypogammaglobulinaemia remains uncertain. B-cell dysfunction often arises early in the disease course and before extensive tumour infiltration of the bone marrow. Thus physical competition for microenvironmental niches able to support B-cell function does not appear to be a satisfactory explanation.

Dilution of the normal B-cell pool due to malignant B-cell expansion could still be a possibility (Kurec & Davey 1987). Aberrant signalling between T and B cells involving the Fas/FasL interaction may also be part of the explanation. B-CLL tumour cells frequently express FasL and are able to inhibit autologous immunoglobulin production by plasma cells *in vitro* (Sampalo *et al.* 2000). The potential significance of this observation was supported by a direct correlation between the intensity of the inhibitory effect *in vitro* and the serum IgG level exhibited by the patient. A further mechanism relates to CD40L expression on activated T cells which is critical in the activation of B cells through CD40 and leads to immunoglobulin class switching and the generation of the IgG isotype. In patients with B-CLL the presence of large numbers of tumour cells expressing CD40 leads to rapid down regulation of CD40L on activated T cells, probably through receptor down-modulation (Cantwell *et al.* 1997). One appealing aspect of this theory is that patients with B-CLL share clinical features in common with children born with inherited defects of the CD40L gene. Finally, direct lysis of B cells and impaired 'help' for antibody production has been observed after culture with T-cell subpopulations isolated from patients (Kaplanski *et al.* 1992; Hersey *et al.* 1980).

Cellular immunity

T cells are the major regulatory and effector cells of the adaptive immune response and there are many reports of T-cell abnormalities in patients with B-CLL (Scrivener *et al.* 2003; Frolova *et al.* 1995; Velardi *et al.* 1985; Herrmann *et al.* 1983). A summary

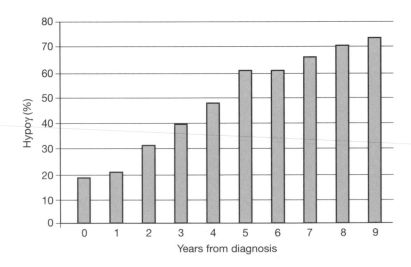

Figure 10.2 Cumulative incidence of hypogammaglobulinaemia in an untreated cohort of patients with B-CLL (based on Rozman 1988).

of the data would suggest that patients exhibit a reduction in the naïve T-cell pool in association with an increase in terminally differentiated memory cells (Briggs *et al.* 1990; Totterman *et al.* 1989). An accumulation of clonally expanded T cells has also been documented (Wen *et al.* 1990). These features resemble an acceleration of the 'immune senescence' that is seen with normal ageing and would suggest an impaired ability to initiate immune responses. This is supported by functional defects in immunity in these patients (see below).

There has been considerable debate concerning the relationship between the B-cell tumour clone and the T-cell repertoire. A tumour-specific T-cell response may play a role in controlling disease progression but such an antigenic specificity has been difficult to demonstrate with a high degree of confidence (Gitelson *et al.* 2003). In contrast, other authors have suggested that T cells may play a role in the maintenance of the B-cell clone and the potential utility of cyclosporin as a therapeutic agent in B-CLL would tend to support this view (Bergui *et al.* 1994). However, notwithstanding a potential tumour-specific T-cell response, it is likely that pathogen-specific immune responses are the major cause of the alterations in T-cell phenotype that are seen in patients with B-CLL. The immune response to cytomegalovirus (CMV) leads to very large expansions of CD4$^+$ and CD8$^+$ T cells that can distort the complete T-cell repertoire (see below). Indeed, it is likely that many of the features of the T-cell repertoire in B-CLL are actually reactive rather than a primary consequence of the disease process.

The immune response to CMV in patient with B-CLL

The absolute T-cell count in peripheral blood is frequently raised in patients with B-CLL (Mackus *et al.* 2003; De Paoli *et al.* 1984). However, when patients are divided into those who have been infected with CMV (and are therefore CMV seropositive) and those who remain CMV seronegative it is clear that this increment in T-cell number is seen predominantly in the CMV seropositive group. Such an effect of CMV seropositivity on T-cell repertoire is seen in many cohorts including the elderly, patients recovering from an allogeneic stem-cell transplant and those with rheumatoid arthritis. The reason for this effect is that CMV is never eradicated from a host after initial infection but remains latent as a consequence of a sustained cellular immune response directed against viral proteins. The magnitude of this response increases with age and as a result of immune suppression. Viraemia is a potent stimulus to the T-cell immune response and it seems likely that episodes of sub-clinical viraemia are the explanation for the increased levels of immunity in patients who are immunosuppressed. The CMV-specific T-cell response is increased in patients with B-CLL compared with an age-matched control group. The CD8$^+$ response is characterised by the accumulation of many effector memory cells with a phenotype (CD27$^-$ CD28$^-$ CD57$^+$) typical of cells that accumulate in B-CLL patients (Mackus *et al.* 2003). The CD4$^+$ T-cell response shows a similar expansion although to a lower level which is typically up to 10% of the total CD4$^+$ T-cell repertoire. These populations are frequently clonal and are the likely explanation for clonal T-cell expansions seen in patients with B-CLL.

CMV seropositivity is associated with an increased mortality rate in the very elderly and it is tempting to speculate that it may also be detrimental to patients with B-CLL, possibly as a consequence of deviation of the immune response away from control of heterologous infection. It is certainly true that the ability of B-CLL patients to respond to influenza vaccine can be correlated with the level of naïve CD4$^+$CD45RA$^+$ T cells (Marotta *et al.* 1998). However, there are currently no data to suggest that CMV seropositivity is a risk factor for increased morbidity or mortality in patients with B-CLL.

Immunosuppression as a consequence of treatment for B-CLL

Clinical experience indicates that patients with B-CLL suffer from an increasing severity and frequency of infection as their disease progresses. Damage to the immune system which is sustained as a result of the treatment is at least one major reason for this observation. A recent report by Hensel *et al.* (2003) followed 187 patients over a 4-year period and showed that treatment history was the predominant risk factor for infection. Sixty per cent of patients suffered from minor infections, defined as those requiring oral antibiotics or treated as an outpatient, whereas 20% had major infections that required inpatient treatment or intravenous antibiotics. Risk factors for major infection were the number of previous chemotherapy regimens and the haemoglobin concentration. The number of previous chemotherapy regimens was the only risk factor for minor infection and varicella zoster infection.

A major review of infectious episodes in 554 patients who were receiving chlorambucil alone, fludarabine alone or combination therapy demonstrated that fludarabine was associated with more major infections and herpes virus infections than chlorambucil (Morrison *et al.* 2001). However, combination therapy led to a markedly increased infection rate.

Purine analogues such as fludarabine are intensely immunosuppressive and indeed are used widely for this precise reason in conditioning regimes before low-intensity stem-cell transplantation (Samonis & Kontoyiannis 2001). A variety of infections have been reported in patients on fludarabine therapy and measurement of a CD4 count of less than 50 cells/ml is correlated with the incidence of herpes zoster reactivation (Anaissie *et al.* 1998). 2-chlorodeoxyadenosine (2-CDA) therapy is also associated with an increased infection rate (Van Den Neste *et al.* 1996; Betticher *et al.* 1994). Patients with advanced disease who are refractory to fludarabine therapy have an extremely high infection rate. One such cohort had a median survival of 13 months with an average of two hospital admissions for serious infection during this time (Perkins *et al.* 2002). One in eight patients suffered from an episode of viral disease with 4.5% suffering from fungal infection and a similar proportion developing other opportunistic infections.

Treatment with monoclonal antibody specific for CDw52 (Campath-1H, MabCampath-1H®) is a potent lymphocytic agent and an effective therapy for a proportion of patients with advanced disease (Rai & Hallek 2002). However, it is not specific in its action and patients are therefore rendered significantly immunosuppressed after treatment. The CAM211 trial used Campath-1H in patients who were refractory to fludarabine, and 14% of the patient cohort suffered from a viral reactivation (Keating *et al.* 2002). Most of these episodes were CMV reactivation and the use of aciclovir is now recommended for patients treated with this agent. There was also a 12% incidence of opportunistic infection including aspergillus, rhinocerebral mucormycosis and systemic candidiasis. Case reports of fatal adenoviral infection and red cell aplasia secondary to parvovirus have also been reported following Campath-1H (Cavalli-Bjorkman *et al.* 2002; Crowley & Woodcock 2002).

The emergence of CMV as a significant viral pathogen is almost solely due to the use of Campath-1H antibody. The peak incidence of reactivation is seen at between 2 and 6 weeks after treatment but the frequency of reactivation has varied in the different trials. Osterborg used Campath-1H as first-line therapy and observed one case of CMV pneumonitis out of 9 cases (Osterborg *et al.* 1996). Bowen et al used Campath-1H in patients refractory to fludarabine and reported reactivation in 3 of 7 patients (Bowen *et al.* 1997) although a subsequent trial identified a lower reactivation rate at 15% (Nguyen *et al.* 2002). The stage of disease at which Campath-1H is used is important but the CMV reactivation rate can still approach 10% when used a first-line therapy (Lundin *et al.* 2002). The use of Campath-1H and rituximab in late stage patients led to a CMV reactivation rate of 27% although not all of these patients required treatment (Faderl *et al.* 2003).

Functional assessment of immunity in patients with B-CLL

Skin testing is a useful assay by which to study the activity of the cellular arm of the immune system. Patients with B-CLL exhibit poor recall responses to skin testing with many patients being anergic to challenge (Miller & Karnofsky 1961). This response correlates with the history of treatment with chemotherapy. The response to primary skin challenge is even worse and indicates a profound impairment of antigen presentation (Cone & Uhr 1964). The ability of patients to respond to novel infections in the environment may thus be seriously compromised.

Vaccination is a better means by which to assess immune function. Impaired responses have been documented in many studies. Responses to the inactivated influenza vaccine may be particularly poor (van der Velden *et al.* 2001). In one report, only 63% of patients were able to maintain an effective humoral response for 2 months after vaccination (Gribabis *et al.* 1994). However, other authors have more recently reported greater success (Rapezzi *et al.* 2003) and influenza vaccination should certainly be encouraged in all patients. Serological responses to *Haemophilus* and *Pneumococcus* can be obtained but are achieved more reliably if given in the early phase of disease (Hartkamp *et al.* 2001). The use of conjugate vaccines appears valuable and the introduction of adjuvants may also enhance the level of response (Sinisalo *et al.* 2003).

The management of immunodeficiency in patients with B-CLL

Patient Education

All patients with a diagnosis of B-CLL should be informed that they are at increased risk of infection and should be advised to seek prompt medical attention in the event of the development of a fever or infectious symptoms.

Vaccination

This would appear to be a sensible option in most patients. Most of the vaccines in common usage, such as influenza or pneumococcal vaccine, are inactivated but live attenuated vaccines should not be used in heavily treated patients with advanced disease.

Antibiotic prophylaxis

Antibiotics are commonly employed in patients with B-CLL but there is no evidence base to support their widespread use. Co-trimoxazole should be used for patients receiving therapy with purine analogues. The optimal duration of therapy is uncertain but they should be continued for at least six months and perhaps longer if the total lymphocyte count has not risen beyond $1 \times 10^9/l$. The use of cytokines such as G-CSF may be indicated in patients with profound neutropenia (Vickers 1997).

Anti-viral prophylaxis

The era of highly immunosuppressive chemotherapy has led to the requirement to consider prophylaxis against viral infection. Patients receiving treatment with Campath-1H anti-CD52 monoclonal antibody should receive oral aciclovir or famciclovir (250 mg b.d.) prophylaxis (Keating *et al.* 2002). In addition, they should be monitored on a regular basis for reactivation of cytomegalovirus using an assay such as polymerase chain reaction (PCR) or antigenemia test. Two consecutive positive results are likely to trigger therapeutic use of ganciclovir in most cases although different centres vary in their threshold for instigation of therapeutic anti-viral therapy.

Immunoglobulin replacement therapy

The introduction of immunoglobulin replacement therapy for patients with primary hypogammaglobulinaemia led naturally to its use in patients with B-CLL. Detection of impaired humoral immunity, as determined by hypogammaglobulinaemia, is a relatively straightforward assay in comparison to assessment of T-cell function. This, combined with the relative simplicity of immunoglobulin replacement, has led to several trials of immunoglobulin replacement. The initial studies involved the use of intramuscular immunoglobulin which was both inconvenient to deliver and poorly effective in providing adequate immunoglobulin replacement. A landmark study was that of the co-operative group for intravenous immunoglobulin replacement (IVIG), the results of which were published in 1988 (Bunch 1988). This was a double blind trial of 84 patients in whom the immunoglobulin level was less than 50% of the normal range or who had a history of serious infection. The treatment arm received IVIG at a dose of 400 mg/kg every 3 weeks for 1 year. Analysis showed that IVIG reduced the number of bacterial infections from 42 in the control arm to 23 in the treatment arm ($p < 0.01$) (Figure 10.3). In those patients who completed a year of therapy the reduction was more dramatic from 36 to 14 ($p < 0.001$). There was no difference in the incidence of non-bacterial infection. However, notwithstanding these encouraging results, the cost effectiveness of IVIG therapy came under significant scrutiny. Weeks *et al.* (1991) used a 'decision-analysis technique' to analyse the trial and inferred that IVIG treatment resulted in a loss of quality-adjusted life expectancy when the inconvenience of the treatment was taken into account. If the inconvenience of treatment was ignored, it was estimated that treatment resulted in a gain of 0.8 quality-adjusted days per patient per year of therapy. The cost of a 'quality adjusted life year gained' was a staggering US$6 million.

These observations led clinicians to develop trials in which lower doses of immunoglobulin were administered. Chapel *et al.* (1994) randomised 34 patients to IVIG at doses of either 500 mg/kg or 250 mg/kg every 4 weeks for one year. There

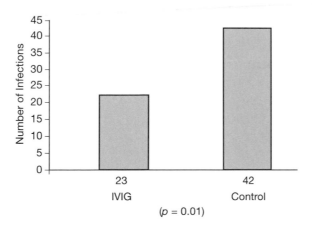

Figure 10.3 Number of infections seen during study duration in patients who received immunoglobulin replacement therapy compared with a control group (Bunch *et al.* 1988).

was no difference in the number or severity of infections in either group. A reduction in the total IVIG dose down to 10 g every 3 weeks also appears effective although only 15 patients were included in this trial (Jurlander *et al.* 1994). Two further trials have confirmed the value of IVIG as doses of 300 mg/kg or 18 g every 3 weeks (Molica *et al.* 1996; Boughton *et al.* 1995).

Unfortunately immunoglobulin replacement remains a relatively time consuming practice and the cost is not inconsiderable. Replacement of 20 g of IVIG on a 3-weekly basis could typically cost around £7000 per year. The result is that at a practical level relatively few patients receive such treatment. The British Committee for Standards in Haematology (BCSH) guidelines suggest that 'patients with hypogammaglobulinaemia and recurrent bacterial infection, especially those in whom prophylactic antibiotics have proved ineffective, should be treated with prophylactic IVIG'. This advice remains appropriate.

Summary

The patient with B-cell chronic lymphocytic leukaemia is at an increased risk of infection throughout the course of their disease. However, the stage of the disease and treatment history are predominant factors in determining both the magnitude of this risk and the nature of the potential pathogens involved. The design of an appropriate management plan for controlling infection must take account of these factors (Figure 10.4).

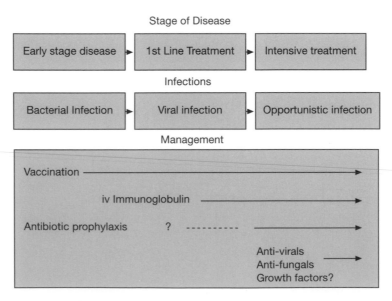

Figure 10.4 Schematic representation of the type of infections that are seen in patients with B-cell at different stages of disease and the management options that are available.

In the early stages of disease bacterial infections are the predominant risk and appropriate vaccinations should be given. At later stages viral infections such as herpes zoster may be witnessed and immunoglobulin replacement therapy or antibiotic prophylaxis may be indicated in selected patients. In the most advanced phase of disease, in which patients are often heavily treated with immunosuppressive drugs, opportunistic infections such as cytomegalovirus or fungal infection may develop and management plans typical of those used for patients undergoing intensive chemotherapy regimens must be developed.

Infection remains one of the most troublesome factors in the management of the patient with B-CLL and is a frequent cause of morbidity and mortality. The pathogenesis of the immunosuppression is not completely understood but involves several factors related both to the primary malignant B-cell expansion and of secondary effects related to infections such as CMV. At present, it is not possible to provide patients with complete protection from infection but clinical approaches based on individual risk are critical in management of the disease.

References

Ahmed, S., Siddiqui, A. K. *et al.* (2003). Pulmonary complications in chronic lymphocytic leukemia. *Cancer* **98**, 1912–1917.

Anaissie, E. J., Kontoyiannis, D. P. *et al.* (1998). Infections in patients with chronic lymphocytic leukemia treated with fludarabine. *Annals of Internal Medicine* **129**, 559–566.

Bergui, L., Gregoretti, M. G. *et al.* (1994). Cyclosporin A in the treatment of B-chronic lymphocytic leukemia (B-CLL). *Leukemia* **8**, 1245–1246.

Betticher, D. C., Fey, M. F. *et al.* (1994). High incidence of infections after 2-chlorodeoxyadenosine (2-CDA) therapy in patients with malignant lymphomas and chronic and acute leukaemias. *Annals of Oncology* **5**, 57–64.

Boggs, D. R. (1960). The cellular composition of inflammatory exudates in human leukemias. *Blood* **15**, 466–475.

Boughton, B. J., Jackson, N. *et al.* (1995). Randomized trial of intravenous immunoglobulin prophylaxis for patients with chronic lymphocytic leukaemia and secondary hypogamma-globulinaemia. *Clinical and Laboratory Haematology* **17**, 75–80.

Bowen, A. L., Zomas, A. *et al.* (1997). Subcutaneous CAMPATH-1H in fludarabine-resistant/relapsed chronic lymphocytic and B-prolymphocytic leukaemia. *British Journal of Haematology* **96**, 617–619.

Briggs, P. G., Kraft, N. *et al.* (1990). T cells and CD45R expression in B-chronic lymphocytic leukemia. *Leukemia Research* **14**, 155–159.

Bunch, C. (1988). Intravenous immunoglobulin for the prevention of infection in chronic lymphocytic leukemia. A randomized, controlled clinical trial. Cooperative Group for the Study of Immunoglobulin in Chronic Lymphocytic Leukemia. *New England Journal of Medicine* **319**, 902–907.

Cantwell, M., Hua, T. *et al.* (1997). Acquired CD40-ligand deficiency in chronic lymphocytic leukemia. *Nature Medicine* **3**, 984–989.

Cavalli-Bjorkman, N., Osby, E. *et al.* (2002). Fatal adenovirus infection during alemtuzumab (anti-CD52 monoclonal antibody) treatment of a patient with fludarabine-refractory B-cell chronic lymphocytic leukemia. *Medical Oncology* **19**, 277–280.

Chapel, H., Dicato, M. *et al.* (1994). Immunoglobulin replacement in patients with chronic lymphocytic leukaemia: a comparison of two dose regimes. *British Journal of Haematology* **88**, 209–212.

Chapel, H. M. & Bunch, C. (1987). Mechanisms of infection in chronic lymphocytic leukemia. *Seminars in Hematology* **24**, 291–296.

Cone, L. & Uhr, J. W. (1964). Immunological Deficiency Disorders Associated with Chronic Lymphocytic Leukemia and Multiple Myeloma. *Journal of Clinical Investigation* **43**, 2241–2248.

Copson, E. R., Ellis, B. A. *et al.* (1994). IgG subclass levels in patients with B cell chronic lymphocytic leukaemia. *Leukemia & Lymphoma* **14**, 471–473.

Crowley, B. & Woodcock, B. (2002). Red cell aplasia due to parvovirus b19 in a patient treated with alemtuzumab. *British Journal of Haematology* **119**, 279–280.

De Paoli, P., Molaro, G. L. *et al.* (1984). Peripheral blood and bone marrow lymphocytes of B chronic lymphocytic leukaemia patients. *Bollettino Dell'istituto Sieroterapico Milanese* **63**, 534–536.

Eftekhari, P., Lassoued, K. *et al.* (1998). Severe respiratory syncytial virus pulmonary infection in a patient treated with fludarabine for chronic lymphocytic leukemia. *Annals of Hematology* **76**, 225–226.

Egerer, G., Hensel, M. *et al.* (2001). Infectious complications in chronic lymphoid malignancy. *Current Treatment Options in Oncology* **2**, 237–244.

Faderl, S., Thomas, D. A. *et al.* (2003). Experience with alemtuzumab plus rituximab in patients with relapsed and refractory lymphoid malignancies. *Blood* **101**, 3413–3415.

Frolova, E. A., Richards, S. J. *et al.* (1995). Immunophenotypic and DNA genotypic analysis of T-cell and NK-cell subpopulations in patients with B-cell chronic lymphocytic leukaemia (B-CLL). *Leukemia & Lymphoma* **16**, 307–318.

Ghosh, K., Sivakumaran, M. *et al.* (1995). Pulmonary tuberculosis after fludarabine for chronic lymphocytic leukaemia. *National Medical Journal of India* **8**, 294–295.

Gitelson, E., Hammond, C. *et al.* (2003). Chronic lymphocytic leukemia-reactive T cells during disease progression and after autologous tumor cell vaccines. *Clinical Cancer Research* **9**, 1656–1665.

Gribabis, D. A., Panayiotidis, P. *et al.* (1994). Influenza virus vaccine in B-cell chronic lymphocytic leukaemia patients. *Acta Haematologica* **91**, 115–118.

Griffiths, H., Lea, J. *et al.* (1992). Predictors of infection in chronic lymphocytic leukaemia (CLL). *Clinical and Experimental Immunology* **89**, 374–377.

Hartkamp, A., Mulder, A. H. *et al.* (2001). Antibody responses to pneumococcal and haemophilus vaccinations in patients with B-cell chronic lymphocytic leukaemia. *Vaccine* **19**, 1671–1677.

Heath, M. E. & Cheson, B. D. (1985). Defective complement activity in chronic lymphocytic leukemia. *American Journal of Hematology* **19**, 63–73.

Hensel, M., Kornacker, M. *et al.* (2003). Disease activity and pretreatment, rather than hypogammaglobulinaemia, are major risk factors for infectious complications in patients with chronic lymphocytic leukaemia. *British Journal of Haematology* **122**, 600–606.

Herrmann, F., Sieber, G. *et al.* (1983). Further evidence for T cell abnormalities in chronic lymphocytic leukaemia of the B cell type. *Clinical and Experimental Immunology* **53**, 109–114.

Hersey, P., Wotherspoon, J. *et al.* (1980). Hypogammaglobulinaemia associated with abnormalities of both B and T lymphocytes in patients with chronic lymphatic leukaemia. *Clinical and Experimental Immunology* **39**, 698–707.

Itala, M., H. Helenius, H. *et al.* (1992). Infections and serum IgG levels in patients with chronic lymphocytic leukemia. *European Journal of Haematology* **48**, 266–270.

Jim, R. T. & Reinhard E. H. (1956). Agammaglobulinemia and chronic lymphocytic leukemia. *Annals of Internal Medicine* **44**, 790–796.

Jurlander, J., Geisler, C. H. *et al.* (1994). Treatment of hypogammaglobulinaemia in chronic lymphocytic leukaemia by low-dose intravenous gammaglobulin. *European Journal of Haematology* **53**, 114–118.

Kaplanski, G., Seidel-Farnarier, C. *et al.* (1992). "NK-like" T cytotoxicity against B lymphocytes in a hypogammaglobulinemic patient. *Immunological Investigations* **21**, 601–612.

Katrinakis, G., Kyriakou, D. *et al.* (1995). Evidence for involvement of activated CD8+/HLA-DR+ cells in the pathogenesis of neutropenia in patients with B-cell chronic lymphocytic leukaemia. *European Journal of Haematology* **55**, 33–41.

Katrinakis, G., Kyriakou, D. *et al.* (1996). Defective natural killer cell activity in B-cell chronic lymphocytic leukaemia is associated with impaired release of natural killer cytotoxic factor(s) but not of tumour necrosis factor-alpha. *Acta Haematologica* **96**, 16–23.

Keating, M. J., Flinn, I. *et al.* (2002). Therapeutic role of alemtuzumab (Campath-1H) in patients who have failed fludarabine: results of a large international study. *Blood* **99**, 3554–3361.

Kimby, E., Mellstedt, H. *et al.* (1989). Differences in blood T and NK cell populations between chronic lymphocytic leukemia of B cell type (B-CLL) and monoclonal B-lymphocytosis of undetermined significance (B-MLUS). *Leukemia* **3**, 501–504.

Kurec, A. S. & Davey, F. R. (1987). Impaired synthesis of immunoglobulin in patients with chronic lymphocytic leukemia. *American Journal of Hematology* **25**, 131–142.

Lacombe, C., Gombert, J. *et al.* (1999). Heterogeneity of serum IgG subclass deficiencies in B chronic lymphocytic leukemia. *Clinical Immunology* **90**, 128–132.

Lundin, J., Kimby, E. *et al.* (2002). Phase II trial of subcutaneous anti-CD52 monoclonal antibody alemtuzumab (Campath-1H) as first-line treatment for patients with B-cell chronic lymphocytic leukemia (B-CLL). *Blood* **100**, 768–773.

Mackus, W. J., Frakking, F. N. *et al.* (2003). Expansion of CMV-specific CD8+CD45RA+CD27- T cells in B-cell chronic lymphocytic leukemia. *Blood* **102**, 1057–1063.

Marotta, G., Bucalossi, A. *et al.* (1998). CD4+/CD45RA+ 'naive' T cells and immunological response to influenza virus vaccine in B-cell chronic lymphocytic leukaemia patients. *Acta Haematologica* **99**, 18–21.

Melzer, M., Colbridge, M. *et al.* (1998). Cryptococcosis: an unusual opportunistic infection complicating B cell lymphoproliferative disorders. *Journal of Infection* **36**, 220–222.

Miller, D. G. & Karnofsky, D. A. (1961). Immunologic factors and resistance to infection in chronic lymphatic leukemia. *American Journal of Medicine* **31**, 748–757.

Molica, S., Levato, D. *et al.* (1993). Infections in chronic lymphocytic leukemia. Analysis of incidence as a function of length of follow-up. *Haematologica* **78**, 374–377.

Molica, S., Musto, P. *et al.* (1996). Prophylaxis against infections with low-dose intravenous immunoglobulins (IVIG) in chronic lymphocytic leukemia. Results of a crossover study. *Haematologica* **81**, 121–126.

Morra, E., Nosari, A. *et al.* (1999). Infectious complications in chronic lymphocytic leukaemia. *Haematological Cell Therapy* **41**, 145–151.

Morrison, V. A., Rai, K. R. *et al.* (2001). Impact of therapy with chlorambucil, fludarabine, or fludarabine plus chlorambucil on infections in patients with chronic lymphocytic leukemia: Intergroup Study Cancer and Leukemia Group B 9011. *Journal of Clinical Oncology* **19**, 3611–3621.

Nguyen, D. D., Cao, T. M. *et al.* (2002). Cytomegalovirus viremia during Campath-1H therapy for relapsed and refractory chronic lymphocytic leukemia and prolymphocytic leukemia. *Clinical Lymphoma* **3**, 105–110.

Osterborg, A., Fassas, A. S. *et al.* (1996). Humanized CD52 monoclonal antibody Campath-1H as first-line treatment in chronic lymphocytic leukaemia. *British Journal of Haematology* **93**, 151–153.

Perkins, J. G., Flynn, J. M. *et al.* (2002). Frequency and type of serious infections in fludarabine-refractory B-cell chronic lymphocytic leukemia and small lymphocytic lymphoma: implications for clinical trials in this patient population. *Cancer* **94**, 2033–2039.

Rai, K. & Hallek, M. (2002). Future prospects for alemtuzumab (MabCampath). *Medical Oncology* **19** (Suppl.), S57–S63.

Rapezzi, D., Sticchi, L. *et al.* (2003). Influenza vaccine in chronic lymphoproliferative disorders and multiple myeloma. *European Journal of Haematology* **70**, 225–230.

Robertson, T. I. (1990). Complications and causes of death in B cell chronic lymphocytic leukaemia: a long term study of 105 patients. *Australian and New Zealand Journal of Medicine* **20**, 44–50.

Rozman, C., Montserrat, E. *et al.* (1988). Serum immunoglobulins in B-chronic lymphocytic leukemia. Natural history and prognostic significance. *Cancer* **61**, 279–283.

Samonis, G. & Kontoyiannis, D. P. (2001). Infectious complications of purine analog therapy. *Current Opinion in Infectious Diseases* **14**, 409–413.

Sampalo, A., Navas, G. *et al.* (2000). Chronic lymphocytic leukemia B cells inhibit spontaneous Ig production by autologous bone marrow cells: role of CD95–CD95L interaction. *Blood* **96**, 3168–3174.

Scrivener, S., R. V. Goddard, *et al.* (2003). Abnormal T-cell function in B-cell chronic lymphocytic leukaemia. *Leukemia & Lymphoma* **44**, 383–389.

Shvidel, L., Vorst, E. *et al.* (1998). Complement values in B chronic lymphocytic leukemia: prognostic significance and correlation with cell maturation stage. *Leukemia* **12**, 635–636.

Sinisalo, M., Aittoniemi, J. *et al.* (2003). Vaccination against infections in chronic lymphocytic leukemia. *Leukemia & Lymphoma* **44**, 649–652.

Sorskaar, D., Forre, O. *et al.* (1988). Natural killer cells in chronic leukemia. Function and markers. *International Archives of Allergy and Applied Immunology* **87**, 159–164.

Sudhoff, T., Arning, M. *et al.* (1997). Prophylactic strategies to meet infectious complications in fludarabine-treated CLL. *Leukemia* **11** (Suppl. 2), S38–S41.

Totterman, T. H., Carlsson, M. *et al.* (1989). T-cell activation and subset patterns are altered in B-CLL and correlate with the stage of the disease. *Blood* **74**, 786–792.

Tsiodras, S., Samonis, G. *et al.* (2000). Infection and immunity in chronic lymphocytic leukemia. *Mayo Clinic Proceedings* **75**, 1039–1054.

Twomey, J. J. (1973). Infections complicating multiple myeloma and chronic lymphocytic leukemia. *Archives of Internal Medicine* **132**, 562–565.

Van Den Neste, E., Delannoy, A. *et al.* (1996). Infectious complications after 2-chlorodeoxyadenosine therapy. *European Journal of Haematology* **56**, 235–240.

van der Velden, A. M., Mulder, A. H. *et al.* (2001). Influenza virus vaccination and booster in B-cell chronic lymphocytic leukaemia patients. *European Journal of Internal Medicine* **12**, 420–424.

Velardi, A., Prchal, J. T. *et al.* (1985). Expression of NK-lineage markers on peripheral blood lymphocytes with T-helper (Leu3+/T4+) phenotype in B cell chronic lymphocytic leukemia. *Blood* **65**, 149–155.

Vickers, M. (1997). Successful use of granulocyte colony-stimulating factor to correct neutropenia in chronic lymphocytic leukaemia. *Clinical and Laboratory Haematology* **19**, 77–78.

Weeks, J. C., Tierney, M. R. *et al.* (1991). Cost effectiveness of prophylactic intravenous immune globulin in chronic lymphocytic leukemia. *New England Journal of Medicine* **325**, 81–86.

Wen, T., Mellstedt, H. *et al.* (1990). Presence of clonal T cell populations in chronic B lymphocytic leukemia and smoldering myeloma. *Journal of Experimental Medicine* **171**, 659–866.

Chapter 11

Autoimmune disease and its management in CLL

Terry J. Hamblin

Introduction

Although the association of autoimmune disease and chronic lymphocytic leukaemia (CLL) is well known, it is often misunderstood. Far from there being a general tendency for patients with CLL to develop autoimmune disease, the only autoimmune conditions commonly seen in CLL are autoimmune haemolytic anaemia (AIHA) and immune thrombocytopenia (ITP). A few other rare conditions occur in CLL more commonly than would be expected, but the common autoimmune diseases such as rheumatoid arthritis, thyroid disease, pernicious anaemia and systemic lupus erythematosus are no commoner in CLL than in age-matched controls.

Autoimmune haemolytic anaemia

Berlin (1951), using the technique of differential agglutination, was the first to show shortened red-cell survival in nine patients with CLL. Wasserman (1955) found haemolytic anaemia to be present in 9 out 58 consecutive patients with CLL, with five out of seven testing positive in the direct antiglobulin test. After this, a series of studies suggested that autoimmune haemolytic anaemia (AIHA) occurs at some time in the course of CLL in between 10–26% of cases (reviewed in Hamblin (2001)).

No one doubts that warm-antibody AIHA is commoner in CLL than in the general population. The highest reported prevalence is 35% (Bergsagel 1967). Conversely, a positive antiglobulin test at diagnosis was found in only 1.8% of patients entered into the French Cooperative Group's CLL1980 and CLL1985 trials (Dighiero 1993). The truth behind the disparity is that the prevalence is closely related to stage and progression. In stable stage A disease, Hamblin *et al.* (1986) found a prevalence of 2.9% compared with 10.5% in stage B and C disease and 18.2% in progressive stage A disease.

Looking at the problem from another point of view, CLL is the commonest known cause of AIHA. In a large series of patients with AIHA, Engelfriet *et al.* (1992) found that 14% were associated with CLL, roughly twice as common as the next known cause, systemic lupus erythematosus. However, in about half the cases of AIHA no cause is found. AIHA is often thought of as a problem with lymphomas generally, but, from Engelfriet's figures it is possible to calculate that AIHA occurs about eight times more commonly in CLL than in other forms of non-Hodgkin's lymphoma, and about two and a half times more commonly than in Hodgkin's disease.

Immune thrombocytopenia

Thrombocytopenia is quite common in CLL. Minot & Buckman (1925) found it in half their patients at presentation and in virtually all those whose white count rose above $175 \times 10^9/l$. Harrington & Arimura (1961) reported seven cases of autoimmune thrombocytopenia occurring in CLL. Ebbe *et al.* (1962) reported five more and suggested that the prevalence of ITP in CLL was 2%; this was endorsed by Hamblin *et al.* (1986) and Dührsen *et al.* (1987). However, in all three series the numbers were small and the reliability of the diagnoses suspect. Diagnosis of ITP in CLL depends on the presence of isolated thrombocytopenia, normal or increased bone marrow megakaryocytes with an excess of early forma, increased mean platelet volume (MPV) and platelet distribution width, and detection of platelet antibodies in the serum or on the platelet membrane.

Unfortunately, tests for platelet antibodies are still unsatisfactory. Hegde *et al.* (1983) found increased levels of platelet associated IgG in three out of ten thrombocytopenia patients with CLL and one out of ten non-thrombocytopenia patients. Even higher rates were found in non-Hodgkin's lymphomas. This test is known to have a high false-positive rate.

Platelet kinetic studies using radiolabelled platelets are seldom performed and in any case demonstrate a shortened survival in splenomegaly. Bone marrows heavily infiltrated with CLL make megakaryocytic numbers difficult to assess. The diagnosis is often made by exclusion and confirmed by response to therapy. The fact that ITP occurs together with AIHA in CLL as Evans' syndrome reinforces the belief that the thrombocytopenia seen in these circumstances has an autoimmune basis. About one-third of patients with ITP secondary to CLL also have a positive direct antiglobulin test, a much higher rate than for primary ITP (Diehl & Ketchum 1998).

Other types of autoimmune disease

Auto-antibodies against the formed elements of the blood may be a special case in CLL. However, apart from immune neutropenia (Killman 1959) and pure red-cell aplasia (Abeloff & Waterbury 1974), Sjøgren's syndrome (Lehner-Netsch *et al.* 1969), nephrotic syndrome (Dathan *et al.* 1974), bullous pemphigoid (Cuni *et al.* 1974) and Graves' disease (Haubenstock & Zalusky 1985) have all been associated with CLL. Reviews by Miller (1962) and Dameshek (1967) also mentioned systemic lupus erythematosus, rheumatoid arthritis, ulcerative colitis, allergic vasculitis and pernicious anaemia. What has been established as true among these allegations?

(a) Autoimmune neutropenia

Neutropenia may occur in CLL because of marrow infiltration or treatment. The well-recognised syndrome of large granular lymphocytic (LGL) leukaemia is regularly associated with neutropenia (Loughran *et al.* 1985), and perhaps some of the earlier reports and impressions mistook this for CLL. A study from Crete (Katrinakis *et al.* 1995) reported higher numbers of CD3$^+$, CD8$^+$ and CD57$^+$ cells in neutropenic patients with CLL and demonstrated that CD8$^+$ cells from neutropenic patients exerted a greater suppressive effect on CFU-GM colony growth than similar cells from non-neutropenic patients. However, this has not been a consistent finding and a recent hypothesis implicates the secretion of high levels of Fas-Ligand in the cause of the neutropenia that is sometimes seen in B-CLL (Lamy & Loughran 1999). Anti-neutrophil antibodies seem to be involved only rarely, if at all.

(b) Pure red-cell aplasia

Like neutropenia, pure red-cell aplasia (PRCA) is a frequent complication of LGL leukaemia; indeed this is probably its commonest cause (Lacy *et al.* 1996). Nevertheless, by 1986 (Chikkappa *et al.* 1986) PRCA had been recognised in as many as 23 cases of B-CLL, and it has subsequently been reported on at least five occasions (Diehl & Ketchum 1998). From their own cases, Chikkappa *et al.* (1986) suggest that the prevalence is about 6%, but this is either an exaggeration borne of underestimating the denominator or the prevalence has been seriously underestimated. In our series, about 1% of our 800 unselected patients with CLL have developed PRCA. It is not possible to estimate how many of these had an autoimmune cause.

(c) Non-haematological autoimmunity

In an elderly population, auto-antibodies are found quite commonly. Hamblin *et al.* (1986) found that a control population of individuals over 60 had tissue-specific auto-antibodies detected by immunofluorescence in 21.5%. In an age-matched series of 195 patients with CLL, the prevalence of auto-antibodies was exactly the same. In this series there were two cases of rheumatoid arthritis, two of cryptogenic cirrhosis, two of immune vasculitis, and one each of pulmonary fibrosis, nephrotic syndrome, polymyositis and polymyalgia rheumatica. Dührsen *et al.* (1987) reported one case each of Graves' disease, Hashimoto's thyroiditis, myasthenia gravis, ankylosing spondylitis and iritis among 104 cases of CLL. Given that patients with active disease are more likely to have a blood test, which would uncover occult CLL; it is probable that all these are chance associations. However, there are three conditions with a considerable literature that should be looked at more closely.

(i) Nephrotic syndrome and glomerulonephritis

It could be argued that nephrotic syndrome occurs more commonly in CLL than would be expected by chance. Dathan *et al.* (1974) reported two cases of CLL who developed nephrotic syndrome caused by an immune complex glomerulonephritis. A Medline search reveals a total of 48 cases, mostly in the form of single case reports. The histological lesion may be either membranous glomerulonephritis or membranoproliferative glomerulonephritis. Although there are two reports of anti-neutrophil cytoplasmic antibodies one of which followed treatment with fludarabine (Dussol *et al.* 1997; Tisler *et al.* 1996), a more likely explanation for the renal disease is the deposition of monoclonal immunoglobulin (sometimes in the form of a cryoglobulin) secreted by the leukaemic cells (Gouet *et al.* 1982; Moulin *et al.* 1992). In most cases the glomerulonephritis remits on successful treatment of the leukaemia.

(ii) Acquired angio-oedema

The syndrome of acquired angio-oedema (AAE) is characterised by late onset of recurrent bouts of angio-oedema and abdominal pain and is caused by an acquired deficiency of the inhibitor of the first component of complement (C1-INH). Type I is associated with lymphoproliferative diseases including CLL and type II with auto-antibodies. The normal C1-INH molecule has a molecular mass (MM) of 105 kDa with a binding site for the serine protease C1s. The auto-antibodies recognize two synthetic peptides (peptides 2 and 3) that span the reactive site of the molecule. A study of six cases of AAE demonstrated that the auto-antibodies were monoclonal whether or not they were associated with a lymphoproliferative disease (He *et al.* 1996). In both types of AAE, a non-functional C1-INH molecule of MM 95 kDa is found in the serum. The mechanism of action of the antibody is to cause or allow the cleavage of the C1-INH molecule and so render it inactive (Chevailler *et al.* 1996).

(iii) Autoimmune blistering skin disease

Oppenheim (1910) probably reported the first patient with CLL and a pemphigoid-like skin disease, although the two patients reported by Sachs (1921) had a more certain diagnosis of CLL. A clear diagnosis of antibody-proven bullous pemphigoid in association with CLL was not achieved until 1974 when Cuni *et al.* described a single case. In their review of the literature they discovered 16 other cases of CLL with either bullous or vesicular skin lesions. Goodnough and Muir (1980) reported the next case 6 years later, but in the same year Laskaris *et al.* (1980) reported two cases of CLL associated with oral pemphigus.

The question as to whether pemphigus or pemphigoid is associated with CLL was resolved when Anhalt *et al.* (1990) described paraneoplastic pemphigus. The clinical features were of painful erosions of the oropharynx, and vermilion borders of the lips that were resistant to conventional treatment. There was a severe pseudomembranous conjunctivitis. Pruritic, polymorphous cutaneous lesions included confluent erythema with skin denudation, and papules on the trunk and extremities forming target lesions with central blistering. Cases had often been previously diagnosed as pemphigus vulgaris or erythema multiforme. Histologically, three elements were observed: suprabasilar intraepithelial acantholysis, necrosis of individual keratinocytes and vacuolar interface change. Immunofluorescence studies revealed the presence in the serum of antibodies that reacted with the intracellular spaces, such as is seen in pemphigus vulgaris or pemphigus foliaceous. However, direct immunofluorescence studies of the skin also demonstrated complement deposition along the basement membrane typical of bullous pemphigoid.

The serum from all the patients immunoprecipitated an identical complex of polypeptides from keratinocyte extracts with MMs ranging from 130 kDa to 250 kDa. These include the antigens that are implicated in both pemphigus and pemphigoid as well as several others. Although it is rare, paraneoplastic pemphigus is a discrete autoimmune blistering skin disease with characteristic clinical features, a pathognomonic pattern of antibody specificity and an association with lymphoid tumours. It may occur in an array of lymphoid tumours, and especially in Castleman's disease, but about 30% of cases occur in CLL (Anhalt & Nousari 1998).

Do tumour cells secrete autoantibody?

Perhaps the simplest explanation for autoimmune disease in CLL would be that the autoantibodies were the product of the tumour. The CLL cell should not be thought of as non-secretory. Using a sensitive radio-immunoassay Stevenson *et al.* (1980) were able to demonstrate secretion of 19S idiotypic IgM in most cases. Baume *et al.* (1994) used a very sensitive immunoblotting technique to find monoclonal immunoglobulins in the sera of 80% of CLLs. However, the light chain type was the same as that of the surface immunoglobulin in only half the cases. Apparently, in CLL serum monoclonal immunoglobulins cannot be assumed to have been produced by the tumour.

There is some evidence that CLL lymphocytes may be committed to produce autoantibodies. Cells from 12/14 CLLs could be induced by stimulation with phorbol ester to secrete IgM that reacted with a variety of autoantigens (Broker *et al.* 1988). Similar polyreactive antibodies have been described by Sthoeger *et al.* (1989). By demonstrating that the antibodies were of the same light chain types as the surface Ig of the CLL cells, they established that the autoantibodies were not the product of contaminating normal B cells. They also demonstrated the production of IgG autoantibodies from CLL cells expressing surface IgG. These findings appeared to give weight to the hypothesis that CLL is derived from a B cell of separate lineage akin to the Ly-1 (CD5) B cell of mice. This hypothesis, though, is increasingly in disrepute (reviewed by Hamblin 2001).

(a) Autoimmune diseases caused by tumour-secreted antibody

Cold agglutination syndrome is the best described disease in which the antibody activity of a monoclonal protein is responsible for the clinical manifestations. The molecular basis for this reaction is now understood. A rat monoclonal antibody, 9G4, raised against the surface IgM of a B cell lymphoma recognised a shared idiotypic determinant on all anti-I or anti-i cold agglutinins (Stevenson *et al.* 1986). Tumour cells from patients with cold agglutination syndrome were immortalised with EBV. The 9G4 positive lines were investigated for the use of immunoglobulin V_H genes and found exclusively to use the V_{4-34} gene (Pascuel *et al.* 1991, 1992). This specificity was retained whether the V_H gene was in germline configuration or showed evidence of somatic mutation. The detailed biochemistry of both the reaction with red cells and with the 9G4 monoclonal has been elucidated (Potter *et al.* 1993).

Cold agglutination syndrome in CLL is rare. Among 78 patients with persistent cold agglutinins reported by Crisp and Pruzanski (1982), six had CLL according to the definition then in use, but so few cases have been published since that it is highly likely that at least some of these cases were of other lymphomas with a greater propensity for secreting large amounts of monoclonal immunoglobulin.

As far as other autoimmune syndromes are concerned, there is little evidence that the autoantibodies are the product of the CLL cell. It is believed that CLL-associated angioedema (He *et al.* 1996) and possibly CLL-associated glomerulonephritis (Gouet *et al.* 1982) may be caused in this way. On the other hand, a recent publication suggests that the anti-230 kDa autoantibody associated with paraneoplastic pemphigus is not synthesized by the CLL cells (Lisery *et al.* 1999). A study by Sikora *et al.* (1979) demonstrated that the monoclonal Ig rescued from CLL cells was not responsible for a concurrent warm antibody AIHA. In contrast, Sthoeger *et al.* (1993) have reported two cases of CLL in whom it was claimed that immunoglobulin eluted from direct antiglobulin positive red cells reacted with anti-κ but not anti-λ antibodies. In addition, the CLL cells produced in culture a monoclonal IgM that reacted with red cells, though more strongly at 4 °C than at 37 °C. Despite this claim, most workers agree that the antibody in AIHA is polyclonal and the product of the residual lymphoid tissue and not of the tumour cells.

Autoimmunity triggered by treatment

Nearly 40 years ago Lewis *et al.* (1966) suggested that haemolysis might be triggered by treatment with X-rays or alkylating agents. Only two such case reports have subsequently appeared in the literature (Catovsky & Foa 1990; Thompson-Moya *et al.* 1989), but among 37 haemolytic episodes in his large series of patients followed for a very long time, Hansen (1973) found only five where treatment with X-rays or alkylating agents had been given in the previous two months. Interestingly, paraneoplastic pemphigus may also be triggered by radiotherapy (Fried *et al.* 1993; Lee *et al.* 1996). Recently, it has become apparent that haemolysis after treatment with the purine analogues is much commoner than after other forms of treatment (Myint *et al.* 1995).

The first report appeared as a letter (Bastion *et al.* 1992). Two cases of AIHA occurred after treatment of CLL with fludarabine, although one had been DAT positive prior to treatment and did not start haemolysing until 5 weeks after the twelfth course of treatment. The association remained in doubt, especially as the MD Anderson Cancer Center group (Houston, Texas), who had most experience in the world of the new drug, argued that the cases they had seen represented the natural prevalence of AIHA in CLL (Di Raimondo *et al.* 1993). Among 112 patients treated with fludarabine they found five patients without pre-existing AIHA who developed haemolysis after between one and six courses, and a further four patients whose pre-existing AIHA deteriorated after fludarabine treatment. In four further patients with pre-existing AIHA fludarabine was given safely.

At the 1994 American Society of Clinical Oncology meeting, Byrd *et al.* (1994) reported a further case and stated that the association had been reported to the US Food and Drug Administration on 30 occasions. A year later Myint *et al.* (1995) reported that of 52 heavily pre-treated patients 12 developed AIHA after between two and six courses of fludarabine. Since then many reports involving more than 100 patients have confirmed the association. The frequency of haemolysis depends on how much previous treatment the patient has received. Only about 2% of patients treated for the first time develop AIHA, compared with about 5% of patients who have received some previous treatment and over 20% of heavily pre-treated patients.

Autoimmune thrombocytopenia may also be triggered by fludarabine. Montillo *et al.* (1994) first reported relapse of CLL associated ITP after exposure to fludarabine. A total of 25 cases of fludarabine related ITP have now been reported (reviewed by Hamblin (2001)). Only one possible case of immune neutropenia has been reported (Stern *et al.* 1999) and three cases of PRCA (Di Raimondo *et al.* 1993; Antich Rojas *et al.* 1997; Leporier *et al.* 1993). Paraneoplastic pemphigus has been reported in five cases (Bazarbachi *et al.* 1995; Braess *et al.* 1997; Littlewood *et al.* 1998). There have been two cases of post-fludarabine glomerulonephritis (Macheta *et al.* 1995; Tisler *et al.* 1996).

The other purine analogues, cladribine and pentostatin are also capable of triggering autoimmune complications (Byrd *et al.* 1995; Robak *et al.* 1997; Hamblin *et al.* 1998; Fleischman & Croy 1995; Chasty *et al.* 1998). Since the best known toxicity of the purine analogues is the profound T-cell suppression, it is interesting to note that treatment with Campath-1 (Otton *et al.* 1999) can trigger autoimmune disease in CLL.

From these observations some general conclusions can be drawn. Most cases of post-fludarabine autoimmunity have occurred in heavily pre-treated patients. Usually patients have previously received an alkylating agent. The complication is severe and often difficult to treat. In many cases it has been fatal. If control is achieved then re-exposure to any of the purine analogues re-triggers the complication. Even alkylating agents may re-trigger it. The recurrence is likely to be even more virulent. Although commonest in CLL, autoimmunity may also be induced in other low-grade lymphoproliferative diseases.

The T-cell hypothesis

Because of the known, almost AIDS-like, CD4 T-cell suppression that occurs after treatment with fludarabine (Boldt *et al.* 1984), Myint *et al.* (1995) it has been suggested that autoimmunity in CLL is caused by loss of T-cell regulatory control of autoreactive T cells.

Autoreactive T cells can readily be identified in the peripheral lymphocyte pool of both humans and mice (Rosekrantz *et al.* 1987). Shevach *et al.* (1998) have identified a population of $CD4^+$ $CD25^+$ T cells that maintain peripheral tolerance. Mice thymectomised on the third day of life develop a wide spectrum of organ-specific autoimmune diseases. Reconstitution of these mice with $CD4^+$ $CD25^+$ T cells from normal mice prevents the development of disease. These cells can also prevent the transfer of disease by autoantigen-specific cloned T cells derived from neonatally thymectomised mice. Elimination of $CD4^+$ $CD25^+$ T cells, which constitute 5–10% of peripheral $CD4^+$ T cells, leads to spontaneous development of various autoimmune diseases (Takahashi *et al.* 1998). They suppress autoreactive T cells by specifically inhibiting the production of IL-2, an action remarkably like that of cyclosporine (Thornton & Shevach 1998). This subset of T cells is very susceptible to killing with chemotherapeutic agents compared with the $CD4^+$ $CD25^-$ subset.

Thymic function declines with age (Winberg & Parkman 1995) and T-cell function is known to be impaired in CLL. Human studies of autoregulatory T cells in CLL have concentrated on the $CD4^+$ $CD45RA^+$ subset. It is not clear whether they represent the same subset as the $CD4^+$ $CD25^+$ subset in the mouse. $CD4^+$ $CD45RA^+$ cells have been shown to be selectively lost in the more advanced stages of CLL, especially in those with autoimmune haemolytic anaemia (Peller & Kaufman 1991).

Treatment of autoimmunity in CLL

There are very few data addressing the problem of how to treat the autoimmune complications of CLL. In general, treatment has been the same as when the disease occurs spontaneously. However, some treatments are less appropriate and there is also the question of whether and how to treat the CLL itself. The possibility that the immunosuppression caused by the disease or its treatment has triggered the autoimmunity has to be weighed against the prospect that treating the disease will eliminate the complication.

(a) Autoimmune haemolytic anaemia

There are no controlled trials of treatment of AIHA secondary to CLL. It is important to note that transfusion of red cells is often vital. Autoimmune destruction of blood cells in CLL is frequently vigorous, especially when triggered by purine analogues, and some patients have died because of the mistaken belief that because transfused cells will also be destroyed by the immune process, they are of no value. It is important also to replenish folic acid. Specific treatment follows what has been established for idiopathic AIHA.

(i) Corticosteroids and cytotoxic drugs

Prednisolone 1 mg/kg for 10–14 days is the standard treatment for acute haemolysis (Damashek & Komninos 1956). The dose is then reduced slowly over the next 3 months. Most patients will respond. The usual steroid side effects, gastric erosions, hypertension and diabetes should be looked for, and especially in immunodeficient patients, prophylaxis against fungal infections should be given. The mode of action of steroids is multifarious and includes decreased lymphocyte proliferation, decreased IL-2 production, decreased T-cell activation and T-helper function, impaired NK function, monocyte maturation and handling of antigen by macrophages, and deficient macrophage chemotaxis (Collins & Newland 1992).

Because most cases occur in progressive CLL, it would be usual to also treat the CLL, either with chlorambucil or fludarabine, but this carries a risk. In patients where the AIHA has been triggered by fludarabine, further exposure to purine analogues (Myint *et al.* 1995; Montillo *et al.* 1995; Vick *et al.* 1998) or even to any other cytotoxic drug may be hazardous (Orchard *et al.* 1998). Conventionally, patients failing to respond to prednisolone, or relapsing when the dose is reduced, are offered azathioprine or cyclophosphamide. In the case of AIHA or ITP complicating CLL, the most appropriate cytotoxic drug should be exhibited.

(ii) Splenectomy

There are very few data on splenectomy in this condition. In a series of 113 splenectomies for AIHA only 4 were for haemolysis secondary to CLL (Coon 1985). The hazards of splenectomy are well known, and are certainly increased in frail, elderly, immunodeficient patients. Nevertheless, it may be lifesaving. In our hands laparoscopic splenectomy extends the possibility of operation to a less healthy population. Patients with AIHA with IgG alone and no complement components on their red cells respond better (Dacie 1975). Before elective splenectomy vaccination against pneumococcus, meningococcus and H. influenza is recommended, and some groups also recommend long-term prophylactic penicillin or equivalent.

(iii) Intravenous immunoglobulin (IvIg)

A review of the literature (Flores *et al.* 1993) details 73 cases of AIHA treated with IvIg. Forty per cent responded. Doses of 0.4g/kg/d for 5 days were effective. Only 18 of the 73 also had CLL. In these reduction of the size of lymph nodes and spleen was noted, response was transient, lasting only 3–4 weeks, but re-treatment was effective (Diehl & Ketchum 1998).

(iv) Cyclosporine

Cyclosporine is used in AIHA when other modalities have failed. When these conditions complicate CLL failure is a common experience, and cyclosporine has been used most frequently in this situation (Ruess-Borst *et al.* 1994; Cortes *et al.* 2001). The dose is 5–8 mg/kg/d, tapering to a maintenance dose of about 3 mg/kg/d. We aim to keep the blood level at about 100 μg/l.

(v) Other treatments

Splenic irradiation may substitute for splenectomy in patients too sick for surgery (Guinet *et al.* 1989). It may be more appropriate where the spleen is very large. Danazol may have a role in steroid sparing, though its use in CLL is unreported (Diehl & Ketchum 1998). Plasma exchange is less fashionable than it was. Although successful in a few reports of idiopathic AIHA, there are no reports in cases secondary to CLL (Diehl & Ketchum 1998). However, the author is aware of one patient so treated who died while attached to the cell separator. Immunoadsorption is an adjunct to plasma exchange where IgG is adsorbed onto a column containing Protein A. At least one patient has been successfully treated in this way (Esa *et al.* 1981). The infusion of vincristine loaded platelets aims at destroying macrophages. One patient whose CLL-related AIHA was unresponsive to other modes of treatment, responded to this heroic measure (Sigler *et al.* 1995).

Autoimmune thrombocytopenia

This complication is so rarely diagnosed that there is next to no guidance in the literature on treatment. It therefore seems wise to follow the Clinical Guidelines of the American Society of Hematology (1997) for the treatment of idiopathic thrombocytopenic purpura and treat the CLL independently as required. Thus, asymptomatic thrombocytopenia should only be treated when the platelet count is less than $30 \times 10^9/l$. Hospitalization should be confined to patients with mucous membrane or other severe bleeding. Conventional dose oral prednisolone is the treatment of choice for those who need any treatment, (those with severe bleeding or a platelet count less than $30 \times 10^9/l$).

Prednisolone is given in the same dose as for AIHA. Patients failing to respond are treated with IvIg 0.4 g/kg/d for 5 days. The response rate is higher than for AIHA. Splenectomy is also more effective than in AIHA with response rates of over 70% in patients unresponsive to steroids (McMillan 1997). Other treatments found to be successful in AIHA may also be tried. Unique to autoimmune thrombocytopenia is treatment with vinca alkaloids. Vincristine 1 mg i.v. weekly × 6 is often effective, but vinblastine has also been used. The drugs may be given as boluses or by slow infusion (Ahn *et al.* 1984).

ITP complicating CLL may be severe causing intractable bleeding such as to constitute a medical emergency. Special measures may need to be taken to control the bleeding. IvIg followed immediately by platelet transfusion (Baumann *et al.* 1986). Alternatively, methylprednisolone 1 g/d i.v. × 3 followed by platelet transfusion may be effective. Tranexamic acid is worth trying.

The management of post-fludarabine autoimmunity

The severity of haemolysis or thrombocytopenia following fludarabine is often extreme and several reports detail fatalities. It is important not to stint on transfusions of red cells or platelets. Patients who develop these complications are often very immunosuppressed and prone to infection. Further immunosuppressive treatment will intensify this risk. We have patients who, despite successful control of the autoimmune complication, have died from cytomegalovirus or aspergillus infections (Myint *et al.* 1995).

Anticipating that the complication will be difficult to control, we move rapidly to secondary treatments. Where steroids have failed we have found success with IvIg and splenectomy, but many of our patients have required cyclosporine and because responses are often delayed we move rapidly to prescribing it.

A special risk is the re-triggering of autoimmunity by re-exposure to fludarabine, cladribine (Myint *et al.* 1995), or pentostatin (Byrd *et al.* 1995). Even chlorambucil may re-trigger the complication (Orchard *et al.* 1998). In a small number of patients it has been possible to reintroduce fludarabine while the patient is maintained on cyclosporine. Whether it is safe to use fludarabine in patients with a positive DAT or evidence of pre-existing AIHA is a vexed question. Certainly some patients have had an exacerbation of their haemolysis or thrombocytopenia when treated this way. Nevertheless, there are reports of both fludarabine and cladribine being used successfully in these circumstances (Montillo *et al.* 1995; Tosti *et al.* 1992). There is little to guide us. Probably purine analogues should be avoided in older, heavily treated patients, and they should always be used with caution.

Pure red-cell aplasia

Treatment for this complication has been reviewed by Diehl & Ketchum (1998). On the basis of literature reports of 41 treatments in 33 patients they recommend instituting treatment to control the CLL since this will be necessary to achieve long term remission of the PRCA. At the same time the PRCA is treated with prednisolone 1 mg/kg/d. If there is no response then cyclosporine is added. The reticulocyte count should increase within 2–3 weeks and the haemoglobin normalises in 1–2 months. At this point the steroid dose can be reduced and stopped. Cyclosporine should be continued for 6–7 months and then gradually withdrawn.

Paraneoplastic pemphigus

This syndrome is frequently fatal: four of the original five patients died (Anhalt *et al.* 1990) and two patients who developed it following fludarabine also succumbed

(Bazarbachi *et al.* 1995; Pott-Hoeck & Hiddemann 1995). One patient has survived post-fludarabine paraneoplastic pemphigus after having been treated with prednisolone 500 mg/d, cyclophosphamide 100 mg/d for several weeks together with IvIg 120 mg over the first 3 days (Braess *et al.* 1997). Other patients with a similar syndrome, unrelated to malignancy, have responded to IvIg (Meir *et al.* 1993; Mohr *et al.* 1995). Four patients have responded to the combination of high dose steroids and cyclosporine or cyclophosphamide, although one later died from sepsis (Littlewood *et al.* 1998; Gergely *et al.* 2003). Rituximab has also been successful in treating such cases (Heizmann *et al.* 2001).

Rapidly progressive glomerulonephritis

Treatment for glomerulonephritis has to involve intense immunosuppression with high-dose intravenous methylprednisolone and cyclophosphamide. Plasma exchange has a role in those cases that present with renal failure requiring dialysis (Levy & Pusey 1997). Aggressive immunosuppression has the added benefit of suppressing the CLL. It is moot whether control of the CLL or control of the autoimmune process is responsible for the beneficial effect of such treatment.

Acquired angioedema

Treatment of this disorder has been recently reviewed by Markovic *et al.* (2000). They recommend treatment of the CLL as the most important element of the management. Otherwise, the androgens, stanozolol and danazol, have been widely used for both the hereditary and acquired form of the disease and are generally successful. They act by increasing the production of C1 esterase inhibitor by the liver. Not all patients are happy taking androgenic steroids, and for many years I have been using tranexamic acid 0.5 g three times daily in the hereditary form. It has been uniformly successful and without side effects. In the one patient with the acquired form that I have seen it has been equally as effective.

References

Abeloff, M. D. & Waterbury, M. D. (1974). Pure red cell aplasia and chronic lymphocytic leukemia. *Archives of Internal Medicine* **134**, 721–724.

Ahn, Y. S., Harrington, W. J., Mylvagnam, R., Allen, L. M. & Pall, L. M. (1984). Slow infusion of vinca alkaloids in the treatment of idiopathic thrombocytopenic purpura. *Annals of Internal Medicine* **100**, 192–196.

American Society of Hematology ITP Practice Guideline Panel (1997). Diagnosis and treatment of idiopathic thrombocytopenic purpura: recommendations of the American Society of Hematology. *Annals of Internal Medicine* **126**, 319–326.

Anhalt, G. J., Kim, S. C., Stanley, J. R., Korman, N. J., Jabs, D. A., Kory, M., Izumi, H., Ratrie, H., Mutasim, D., Ariss-Abda, L. & Labib R. S. (1990). Paraneoplastic pemphigus. An autoimmune mucocutaneous disease associated with neoplasia. *New England Journal of Medicine* **323**, 1729–1735.

Anhalt, G. J. & Nousari, H. C. (1998). Paraneoplastic autoimmune syndromes. In *The Autoimmune Diseases*, 3rd edn (ed. N. R. Rose & I. R. Mackay), pp. 795–804. San Diego: Academic Press.

Antich Rojas, J., Balaguer, H. & Cladera, A. (1997). Selective aplasia of the red-cell series after fludarabine administration in a patient with chronic B-cell lymphatic leukaemia. *Sangre (Barcelona)* **42**, 254–256.

Bastion, Y., Coiffier, B., Dumontet, C., Espinouse, D. & Bryon, P. A. (1992). Severe autoimmune hemolytic anaemia in two patients treated with fludarabine for chronic lymphocytic leukaemia. *Annals of Oncology* **3**, 171–172.

Baumann, M. A., Menitove, J. E., Aster, R. H. & Anderson, T. (1986). Urgent treatment of idiopathic thrombocytopenic purpura with single dose gammaglobulin infusion followed by platelet transfusion. *Annals of Internal Medicine* **104**, 808–809.

Bazarbachi, A., Bachelez, H., Dehen, L., Delmer, A., Zittoun, R. & Dubertret, L. (1995). Lethal paraneoplastic pemphigus following treatment of chronic lymphocytic leukaemia with fludarabine. *Annals of Oncology* **6**, 730–731.

Baume, A., Brizard, A., Dreyfus, B. & Preud'homme, J. L. (1994). High incidence of serum monoclonal Igs detected by a sensitive immunoblotting technique in B-cell chronic lymphocytic leukaemia. *Blood* **84**, 1216–1219.

Bergsagel, D. E. (1967). The chronic leukaemias: a review of disease manifestations and the aims of therapy. *Canadian Medical Association Journal* **96**, 1615–1620.

Berlin, R. (1951). Red cell survival studies in normal and leukaemic subjects; latent haemolytic syndrome in leukaemia with splenomegaly – nature of anaemia in leukaemia – effect of splenomegaly. *Acta Medica Scandinavica* (Suppl.) **252, 139**, 1–141.

Boldt, D. H., Van Hoff, D. D., Kuhn, J. G. & Hersh, M. (1984). Effect on human peripheral lymphocytes of the in vivo administration of 9-β-D-arabinofuranosyl-5′-monophosphate (NSC312887) a new purine antimetabolite. *Cancer Research* **44**, 4661–4666.

Braess, J., Reich, K., Willert, S., Strutz, F., Neumann, C., Hiddemann, W. & Wormann, B. (1997). Mucocutaneous autoimmune syndrome following fludarabine therapy for low-grade non-Hodgkin's lymphoma of B-cell type (B-NHL). *Annals of Hematology* **75**, 227–230.

Broker, B. M., Klajman, A., Youinou, P., Jouquan, J., Worman, C. P., Murphy, J., Mackenzie, L., Quarty-Papafio, R., Blaschek, M. & Collins, P. (1988). Chronic lymphocytic leukemia (CLL) cells secrete multispecific autoantibodies. *Journal of Autoimmunity* **1**, 469–481.

Byrd, J. C., Hertler, A. A., Weiss, R. B., Freiman, J., Kweder, S. L. & Diehl, L. F. (1995). Fatal recurrence of autoimmune hemolytic anaemia following pentostatin therapy in a patient with a history of fludarabine-associated hemolytic anaemia. *Annals of Oncology* **6**, 300–301.

Byrd, J. C., Weiss, R. B., Kweeder, S. L. & Deihl, L. F. (1994). Fludarabine therapy with lymphoid malignancies is associated autoimmune hemolytic anaemia. *Proceedings of American Society of Clinical Oncology* **13**, 304a.

Catovsky, D. & Foa, R. (1990). B-cell chronic lymphocytic leukaemia. In *The Lymphoid Leukaemias* (ed. D. Catovsky & R. Foa), pp. 73–112. London: Butterworths.

Chasty, R. C., Myint, H., Oscier, D. G., Orchard, J., Busuttil, D. P., Hamon, M. D., Prentice, A.G. & Copplesone, J. A. (1998). Autoimmune haemolysis in patients with B-CLL treated with chlorodeoxyadenosine (CDA). *Leukemia & Lymphoma* **29**, 391–398.

Chevailler, A., Arlaud, G., Ponard, D., Pernollet, M., Carrere, F., Renier, G., Drouet, M., Hurez, D. & Gardais, J. (1996). C-1-inhibitor binding monoclonal immunoglobulins in three patients with acquired angioneurotic edema. *Journal of Allergy and Clinical Immunology* **97**, 998–1008.

Chikkappa, G., Zarrabi, M. H. & Tsan, M. F. (1986). Pure red cell aplasia in patients with chronic lymphocytic leukaemia. *Medicine (Baltimore)* **65**, 339–351.

Collins, P. W & Newland, A. C. (1992). Treatment modalities of autoimmune blood disorders. *Seminars in Hematology* **29**, 64–74.

Coon, W. W. (1985). Splenectomy in the treatment of hemolytic anaemia. *Archives of Surgery* **120**, 625–628.

Cortes, J., O'Brien, S., Loscertales, J., Kantarjian, H., Giles, F., Thomas, D., Koller, C. & Keating, M. (2001). Cyclosporin A for the treatment of cytopenia associated with chronic lymphocytic leukemia. *Cancer* **92**, 2016–2022.

Crisp, D. & Pruzanski, W. (1982). B-cell neoplasms with homogeneous cold-reacting antibodies (cold agglutinins). *American Journal of Medicine* **72**, 915–922.

Cuni, L. J., Grünwald, H. & Rosner, F. (1974). Bullous pemphigoid in chronic lymphocytic leukaemia with the demonstration of anti-basement membrane antibodies. *American Journal of Medicine* **57**, 987–992.

Dacie, J. V. (1975). Autoimmune hemolytic anaemia. *Archives of Internal Medicine* **135**, 1293–1300.

Dameshek, W. & Komninos, Z. P. (1956). The present status of treatment of autoimmune hemolytic anaemia with ACTH and cortisone. *Blood* **11**, 648–664.

Dameshek, W. (1967). Chronic lymphocytic leukemia – an accumulative disease of immunologically incompetent lymphocytes. *Blood* **29**, 566–584.

Dathan, J. R. E., Heyworth, M. F. & MacIver, A. G. (1974). Nephrotic syndrome in chronic lymphocytic leukaemia. *British Medical Journal* **3**, 655–657.

Diehl, L. F. & Ketchum, L. H. (1998). Autoimmune disease and chronic lymphocytic leukaemia: autoimmune hemolytic anaemia, pure red cell aplasia and autoimmune thrombocytopenia. *Seminars in Hematology* **25**, 80–97.

Dighiero, G. (1993). Hypogammaglobulinemia and disordered immunity in CLL. In: *Chronic Lymphocytic Leukaemia: Scientific Advances and Clinical Developments* (ed. B. Cheson), pp. 167–180. New York: Marcel Dekker.

Di Raimondo, F., Guistolisi, R., Caccio, A. E., O'Broen, S., Kantarjian, H., Robertson, L. B. & Keating, M. J. (1993). Autoimmune hemolytic anaemia in chronic lymphocytic leukaemia patients treated with fludarabine. *Leukaemia & Lymphoma* **11**, 63–68.

Dührsen, U., Augener, W., Zwingers, T. & Brittinger, G. (1987). Spectrum and frequency of autoimmune derangements in lymphoproliferative disorders: analysis of 637 cases and comparison with myeloproliferative diseases. *British Journal of Haematology* **67**, 235–239.

Dussol, B., Brunet, P., Vacher-Coponat, H., Bouabdallah, R., Chetaille, P. & Berland, Y. (1997). Crescentic glomerulonephritis with antineutrophil cytoplasmic antibodies associated with chronic lymphocytic leukaemia. *Nephrology, Dialysis, Transplantation* **12**, 785–786.

Ebbe, S., Wittels, B. & Dameshek, W. (1962). Autoimmune thrombocytopenic purpura ("ITP type") with chronic lymphocytic leukaemia. *Blood* **19**, 23–27.

Engelfriet, C. P., Overbeeke, M. A. M. & von dem Borne, A. E. G. K. (1992). Autoimmune hemolytic anaemia. *Seminars in Hematology* **29**, 3–12.

Esa, E. C., Ray, P. K., Swami, V. K., Iddiculla, A., Rhoades, J. E. Jr, Bassett, J. G., Joseph, R. R. & Cooper, D. R. (1981). Specific immunoadsorption of IgG antibody in a patient with chronic lymphocytic leukaemia and autoimmune hemolytic anaemia. *American Journal of Medicine* **71**, 1035–1040.

Fleischman, R. A. & Croy, D. (1995). Acute onset of severe autoimmune hemolytic anaemia after treatment with 2-chlorodeoxyadenosine for chronic lymphocytic leukaemia. *American Journal of Hematology* **48**, 293.

Flores, G., Cunningham-Rundles, C., Newland, A. C. & Bussel, J. (1993). Efficacy of intravenous immunoglobulin in the treatment of autoimmune hemolytic anaemia: results in 73 patients. *American Journal of Hematology* **44**, 237–242.

Fried, R., Lynfield, Y., Vitale, P. & Anhalt, G. (1993). Paraneoplastic pemphigus appearing as a bullous pemphigoid eruption after palliative radiation therapy. *Journal of the American Academy of Dermatology* **29**, 815–817.

Gergely, L., Varoczy, L., Vadasz, G., Remenyik, E. & Illes, A. (2003). Successful treatment of B cell chronic lymphocytic leukemia-associated severe paraneoplastic pemphigus with cyclosporin A. *Acta Haematologica* **109**, 202–205.

Goodnough, L. T. & Muir, A. (1980). Bullous pemphigoid as a manifestation of chronic lymphocytic leukaemia. *Archives of Internal Medicine* **140**, 1526–1527.

Gouet, D., Marechaud, R., Touchard, G., Abadie, J. C., Pourrat, O. & Sudre, Y. (1982). Nephrotic syndrome associated with chronic lymphocytic leukaemia. *Nouvelle Presse Medicale* **11**, 3047–3049.

Guinet, M. J., Liew, K. H., Quong, G. G. & Cooper, I. A. (1989). A study of splenic irradiation in chronic lymphocytic leukaemia. *International Journal of Radiation Oncology, Biology, Physics* **16**, 225–229.

Hamblin, T. J. (2001). Autoimmune disease and its management in chronic lymphocytic leukaemia. In *Chronic Lymphoid Leukemias*, 2nd edition (ed. B. D. Cheson), pp. 435–458. New York: Marcel Dekker.

Hamblin, T. J., Orchard, J. A., Myint, H. & Oscier, D. G. (1998). Fludarabine and hemolytic anaemia in chronic lymphocytic leukaemia. *Journal of Clinical Oncology* **16**, 3209.

Hamblin, T. J., Oscier, D. G. & Young, B. J. (1986). Autoimmunity in chronic lymphocytic leukaemia. *Journal of Clinical Pathology* **39**, 713–716.

Hansen, M. M. (1973). Chronic lymphocytic leukaemia: clinical studies based on 189 cases followed for a long time. *Scandinavian Journal of Haematology* **18** (Suppl. 1), 1–282.

Harrington, W. J. & Arimura, G. (1961). Immune reactions of platelets. In *Blood Platelets* (ed. S. A. Johnson, R. W. Monto, J. W. Rebuck & R. C. Horn), pp. 39–84. Boston: Little, Brown.

Haubenstock, A. & Zalusky, R. (1985). Autoimmune hyperthyroidism and thrombocytopenia in a patient with chronic lymphocytic leukemia. *American Journal of Hematology* **19**, 281–283.

He, S., Tsang, S., North, J., Chohan, N., Sim, R. B. & Whaley, K. (1996). Epitope mapping of C1 inhibitor autoantibodies from patients with acquired C1 inhibitor deficiency. *Journal of Immunology* **156**, 2009–2013.

Hegde, U. M., Williams, K., Devereux, S., Bowes, A., Powell, D. & Fisher, D. (1983). Platelet associated IgG and immune thrombocytopenia in lymphoproliferative and autoimmune disorders. *Clinical and Laboratory Haematology* **5**, 9–15.

Heizmann, M., Itin, P., Wernli, M., Borradori, L. & Bargetzi, M. J. (2001). Successful treatment of paraneoplastic pemphigus in follicular NHL with rituximab: report of a case and review of treatment for paraneoplastic pemphigus in NHL and CLL. *American Journal of Hematology* **66**, 142–144.

Katrinakis, G., Kyriakou, D., Alexandrakis, M., Sakellariou, D., Foudoulakis, A. & Eliopoulos, G. D. (1995). Evidence for involvement of activated CD8+/HLA-DR+ cells in the pathogenesis of neutropenia in patients with B-cell chronic lymphocytic leukaemia. *European Journal of Haematology* **55**, 33–41.

Killman, S.-Å. (1959). Auto-aggressive leukocyte agglutinins in leukaemia and chronic leukopenia. *Acta Medica Scandinavica* **163**, 207–222.

Lacy, M. Q., Kurtin, P. J. & Tefferi, A. (1996). Pure red cell aplasia: association with large granular lymphocytic leukaemia and the prognostic value of cytogenetic abnormalities. *Blood* **87**, 3000–3006.

Lamy, T. & Loughran, T. P. (1999). Current concepts: large granular lymphocyte leukaemia. *Blood Reviews* **13**, 230–240.

Laskaris, G. C., Papavasilou, S. S., Bovopoulou, O. D., Nicolis, G. D. (1980). Association of oral pemphigus with chronic lymphocytic leukaemia. *Oral Surgery Oral Medicine Oral Pathology* **50**, 244–249.

Lehner-Netsch, G., Barry, A. & Delage, J. M. (1969). Leukaemias and autoimmune diseases: Sjøgren's syndrome and hemolytic anaemia associated with chronic lymphocytic leukaemia. *Canadian Medical Association Journal* **100**, 1151–1154.

Leporier, M., Reman, O. & Troussard, X. (1993). Pure red cell aplasia with fludarabine for chronic lymphocytic leukaemia. *The Lancet* **342**, 555.

Levy, J. B. & Pusey, C. D. (1997). Still a role for plasma exchange in rapidly progressive glomerulonephritis? *Journal of Nephrology* **10**, 7–13.

Lewis, F. B., Schwarz, R. S. & Damashek, W. (1966). X-irradiation and alkylating agents as possible trigger mechanisms in autoimmune complications of malignant lymphoproliferative diseases. *Clinical and Experimental Immunology* **1**, 3–11.

Lee, M. S., Kossard, S., Ho, K. K., Barnetson, R. S. & Ravich, R. B. (1995). Paraneoplastic pemphigus triggered by radiotherapy. *Australasian Journal of Dermatology* **36**, 206–210.

Lisery, L., Cambazard, F., Rimokh, R., Ghohestani, R., Magaud, J. P., Gaudillere, A., Perot, J.L., Berard, F., Claudy, A., Guyotat, D., Schmitt, D. & Vincent, C. (1999). Bullous pemphigoid associated with chronic B-cell lymphatic leukaemia: the anti-230-kDa autoantibody is not synthesized by leukemic cells. *British Journal of Dermatology* **141**, 155–157.

Littlewood, T. J., Gooplu, C., Lyon, C. C., Carmichael, A. J., Oliwiecki, S., McWhannel, A., Amagai, N., Nishikawa, T., Hashimoto, T. & Wojnarowska, F. (1998). Paraneoplastic pemhigus – an association with fludarabine. *Blood* **92** (Suppl. 1), 280b (abstract 4207).

Loughran, T. P., Kardin, M. E., Starkebaum, G., Abkowitz, J. L., Clark, E. A., Disteche, C., Lum, L. G. & Slichter, S. J. (1985). Leukaemia of large granular lymphocytes: association with clonal chromosomal abnormalities and autoimmune neutropenia, thrombocytopenia, and hemolytic anaemia. *Annals of Internal Medicine* **102**, 169–175.

Macheta, M. P., Parapia, L. A. & Gouldesbrough, D. R. (1995). Renal failure in a patient with chronic lymphocytic leukaemia treated with fludarabine *Journal of Clinical Pathology* **48**, 181–182.

McMillan, R. (1997).Therapy for adults with refractory chronic immune thrombocytopenic purpura. *Annals of Internal Medicine* **126**, 307–314.

Marcovic, S. N., Inwards, D. J., Frigas, E. A. & Phyliky. R. P. (2000). Acquired C1 esterase inhibitor deficiency. *Annals of Internal Medicine* **132**, 144–150.

Meir, F., Sonnichsen, K., Schaumburg-Lever, G., Dopfer, R. & Rassner, G. (1993). Epidermolysis bullosa acquisita: efficiency of high dose intravenous immunoglobulins. *Journal of the American Academy of Dermatology* **29**, 334–337.

Miller, D. G. (1962). Patterns of immunological deficiency in lymphomas and leukemias. *Annals of Internal Medicine* **57**, 703–715.

Minot, G. R., & Buckman, T. E. (1925). The blood platelets in the leukaemias. *American Journal of Medical Science* **169**, 477–485.

Mohr, C., Sunderkottewr, C., Hildebrand, A., Biel, K., Rutter, A., Rutter, G., Luger, T. & Kolde, G. (1995). Successful treatment of epidermolysis bullosa acquisita using intravenous immunoglobulins. *British Journal of Dermatology* **132**, 824–826.

Montillo, M., Tedeschi, A., Delfini, C., Olivieri, A., D'Adamo, F. & Leoni, P. (1995). Effectiveness of fludarabine in advanced B-cell chronic lymphocytic leukaemia. *Tumori* **81**, 419–423.

Montillo, M., Tedeschi, A. & Leoni, P. (1994). Recurrence of autoimmune thrombocytopenia after treatment with fludarabine in a patient with chronic lymphocytic leukaemia. *Leukemia & Lymphoma* **15**, 187–188.

Moulin, B., Ronco, P. M., Mougenot, B., Francois, A., Fillastre, J. P. & Mignon, F. (1992). Glomerulonephritis in chronic lymphocytic leukaemia and related B cell lymphomas. *Kidney International* **42**, 127–135.

Myint, H., Copplestone, J. A., Orchard, J., Craig, V., Curtis, D., Prentice, A. G., Hamon, M. D., Oscier, D. G. & Hamblin, T. J. (1995). Fludarabine-related autoimmune haemolytic anaemia in patients with chronic lymphocytic leukaemia. *British Journal of Haematology* **91**, 341–344.

Oppenheim, M. (1910). Verhandlungen Der Weiner Dermatologischen Gesellschaft. *Archive Dermatologie Syphiligrasse* **101**, 379–382.

Orchard, J., Bolam, S., Myint, H., Oscier, D. G. & Hamblin T. J. (1998). In patients with lymphoid tumours recovering from the autoimmune complications of fludarabine, relapse may be triggered by conventional chemotherapy. *British Journal of Haematology* **102**, 1112–1113.

Otton, S. H., Turner, D. L., Frewin, R., Davies, S. V. & Johnson, S. A. (1999). Autoimmune thrombocytopenia after treatment with Campath 1H in a patient with chronic lymphocytic leukaemia *British Journal of Haematology* **106**, 261–262.

Pascual, V., Victor, K., Lelsz, D., Spellerberg, M. B., Hamblin, T. J., Thompson, K. M., Randen, I., Natvig, J., Capra, J. D. & Stevenson, F. K. (1991). Nucleotide sequence analysis of the V regions of two IgM cold agglutinins. Evidence that the V_H4-21 gene segment is responsible for the major cross-reactive idiotype. *Journal of Immunology* **146**, 4385–4391.

Pascual, V., Victor, K., Spellerberg, M., Hamblin, T. J., Stevenson, F. K. & Capra, J. D. (1992). VH restriction among human cold agglutinins: The VH4-21 gene segment is required to encode anti-I and anti-i specificities. *Journal of Immunology* **149**, 2337–2344.

Peller, S. & Kaufman, S. (1991).Decreased CD45RA T cells in B-cell chronic lymphatic leukaemia patients: correlation with disease stage. *Blood* **78**, 1569–1573.

Pisciotta, A. V. & Hirschboeck, J. S. (1957). Therapeutic considerations in chronic lymphocytic leukaemia. *Archives of Internal Medicine* **99**, 334–335.

Potter, K. N., Li, Y., Pascuel, V., Williams, R. C., Byres, L. A., Spellerberg, M., Stevenson, F. K. & Capra J. D. (1993). Molecular characterization of a cross-reactive idiotope on human immunoglobulins utilizing the V_H4-21 gene segment. *Journal of Experimental Medicine* **178**, 1419–1428.

Pott-Hoeck, C. & Hiddemann, W. (1995). Purine analogues in the treatment of low grade lymphomas and chronic lymphocytic leukaemias. *Annals of Hematology* **6**, 421–433.

Ruess-Borst, M. A., Waller, H. D., Muller, C. A. (1994). Successful treatment of steroid resistant hemolysis in chronic lymphocytic leukaemia with cyclosporine A. *American Journal of Hematology* **9**, 357–359.

Robak, T., Blasinska-Morawiec, M., Krykowski, E., Hellmann, A. & Konopka, L. (1997). Autoimmune haemolytic anaemia in patients with chronic lymphocytic leukaemia treated with 2-chlorodeoxyadenosine (cladribine). *European Journal of Haematology* **58**, 109–113.

Rosenkrantz, K., Dupont, B. & Flomenberg, N. (1987). Relevance of autocytotoxic and autoregulatory lymphocytes in the maintenance of self tolerance. *Concepts in Immunopathology* **4**, 22–41.

Sachs, O. (1921). Ueber Pemphigoide Hauteruption in Einem Falle von Lymphatischer Leukaemie. *Wien Klinikum Wochenschraft* **34**, 317

Shevach, E. M., Thornton, A. & Suri-Payer, E. (1998). T lymphocyte-mediated control of autoimmunity. *Novartis Foundation Symposium* **215**, 200–211.

Sigler, E., Shtalrid, M., Goland, S., Stoeger, Z. M. & Berrebi, A. (1995). Intractable acute autoimmune hemolytic anaemia in B-cell chronic lymphocytic leukaemia successfully treated with vincristine loaded platelet infusion. *American Journal of Hematology* **50**, 313–315.

Sikora, K., Kirkorian, J. & Levy, R. (1979). Monoclonal immunoglobulin rescued from a patient with chronic lymphocytic leukaemia and autoimmune hemolytic anaemia. *Blood* **54**, 513–518.

Stern, S. C., Shah, S. & Costello, C. (1999). Probable autoimmune neutropenia induced by fludarabine treatment for chronic lymphocytic leukaemia. *British Journal of Haematology* **106**, 836–837.

Stevenson, F. K., Hamblin, T. J., Stevenson, G. T. & Tutt, A. (1980). Extracellular idiotypic immunoglobulin arising from human leukaemia B lymphocytes. *Journal of Experimental Medicine* **152**, 1484–1496.

Stevenson, F. K., Wrightham, M., Glennie, M. J., Jones, D. B., Cattan, T., Feizi, T., Hamblin, T. J. & Stevenson, G. T. (1986). Antibodies to shared idiotypes as agents for analysis and therapy for human B cell tumours. *Blood* **68**, 430–436.

Sthoeger, Z. M., Stoeger, D., Shtalrid, M., Sigler, E., Geltner, D. & Berrebi, A. (1993). Mechanism of autoimmune hemolytic anaemia in chronic lymphocytic leukaemia. *American Journal of Hematology* **43**, 259–264.

Sthoeger, Z. M., Wakai, M., Tse, D. B., Viciguerra, V. P., Allen, S. L., Budman, D. R., Lichtman, S. M., Schulman, P., Weiselberg, L. R. & Chiorazzi, N. (1989). Production of autoantibodies by CD5-expressing B lymphocytes from patients with chronic lymphocytic leukaemia. *Journal of Experimental Medicine* **169**, 255–268.

Takahashi, T., Kuniyasu, Y., Toda, M., Sakaguchi, N., Itoh, M., Iwata, M., Shimizu, J. & Sakaguchi, S. (1998). Immunologic self-tolerance maintained by CD25+ CD4+ naturally anergic and suppressive T cells: induction of autoimmune disease by breaking their anergic/suppressive state. *International Immunology* **19**, 1969–1980.

Thompson-Moya, L., Martin, T., Heuft, H.G., Neubaur, A. & Herrmann, R. (1989). Allergic reaction with immune hemolytic anaemia arising from chlorambucil. *American Journal of Hematology* **32**, 230–231.

Thornton, A. M. & Shevach, E. M. (1998). CD4+ CD25+ immunoregulatory T cells suppress polyclonal T cell activation by inhibiting interleukin 2 production. *Journal of Experimental Medicine* **188**, 287–296.

Tisler, A., Pierratos, A. & Lipton, J. H. (1996). Crescentic glomerulonephritis with p-ANCA positivity in fludarabine-treated chronic lymphocytic leukaemia. *Nephrology, Dialysis, Transplantation* **11**, 2306–2308.

Tosti, S., Caruso, R., D'Adamo, F., Picardi, A., Ali-Ege, M., Girelli, G., Mauro, F. R., Marillo, L. & Amadori, S. (1992). Severe autoimmune hemolytic anaemia in a patient with chronic lymphocytic leukaemia responsive to fludarabine responsive treatment. *Annals of Hematology* **65**, 238–239.

Vick, D. J., Byrd, J. C., Beal, C. L. & Chaffin, D. J. (1998). Mixed-type autoimmune hemolytic anaemia following fludarabine treatment in a patient with chronic lymphocytic leukaemia/small cell lymphoma. *Vox Sanguinis* **74**, 122–126.

Videbæk, Aa. (1962). Auto-immune haemolytic anaemia in some malignant systemic diseases. *Acta Medica Scandinavica* **171**, 463–476.

Wasserman, L. R., Stats, D., Schwartz, L. & Fudenberg, H. (1955). Symptomatic and hemopathic hemolytic anaemia. *American Journal of Medicine* **18**, 961–989.

Winberg, K. & Parkman, R. (1995). Age, the thymus and T lymphocytes. *New England Journal of Medicine* **332**, 182–183.

PART 4

Clinical trials and clinical practice guidelines

Chapter 12

Clinical trials on chronic lymphocytic leukaemia in the United Kingdom

Daniel Catovsky, on behalf of the CLL Working Group and the Adult Leukaemia Working Party of the National Cancer Research Institute*

Early MRC trials

Randomised clinical trials on chronic lymphocytic leukaemia (CLL) have been performed in the UK for over 25 years. CLL trials in the late 1970s and 1980s included agents that were already established at the time and not the more recent purine analogues. CLL1 compared chlorambucil, COP (cyclophosphamide, vincristine and prednisolone) and low-dose splenic irradiation. There were no differences in response rates or survival between the arms. Of interest is that the COP combination used, at the beginning, a relatively low dose of cyclophosphamide (125 mg/m^2/day × 5 days). As it was obvious that the responses were low, the dose was doubled in the next series of patients, with improvements in results (Catovsky *et al.* 1991). The question of the correct dose of alkylating agent used in CLL is also relevant to chlorambucil (see below). CLL1 included a question of early or delayed (or no) therapy for Rai stages I/II (Binet A) which, later, with the CLL2A trial, was included in a large meta-analysis of randomised trials of early vs delayed therapy and showed no survival advantage for early intervention with chlorambucil (CLL Trialists' Collaborative Group 1999). CLL2 also compared chlorambucil alone versus chlorambucil plus prednisolone given in monthly courses, which showed no difference in response rate or survival (Catovsky *et al.* 1991). A total of 424 patients in 3 randomised trials (including CLL2) were analysed in the meta-analysis. This overview did not suggest an advantage for adding monthly prednisolone (CLL Trialists' Collaborative Group). This was already obvious, too, in CLL1, which used prednisolone and vincristine as part of COP. It should be noted that all CLL trials in the UK, from CLL1 to the current CLL4, recommend the use of prednisolone in the initial treatment (*ca.* 6 weeks) of Binet stage C patients (Rai III–IV) who have anaemia and/or low platelet counts. Although this use of prednisolone was never tested in a randomised fashion it clearly appears to improve bone marrow function before the introduction of an alkylating agent. Whether this is still necessary with the new regimens using fludarabine is not clear. It is an optional, non-compulsory

*Members of the CLL Working Group during the planning of the LRF-funded CLL4 trial: D. Catovsky (Trial Coordinator), S. Richards (Trial Statistician), A. G. Bosanquet, J. A. Child, T. J. Hamblin, D. W. Milligan, S. Schey, A. G. Smith. Current Chairman of NCRI CLL Working Group: P. Hillmen.

recommendation in CLL4. After six weeks of steroids, patients feel better, platelets and Hb improve, lymph nodes and spleen decrease in size, and the lymphocyte count increases for a while and later drops below the original levels.

Prognostic factors

The analysis of prognostic factors in the UK CLL trials has shown the importance of stage, age, sex and response to therapy (Catovsky *et al.* 1989). The relevance of stage is only significant when the whole population of CLL patients is considered (Figure 12.1). Once established that most patients with stage A do not benefit from early therapy with chlorambucil, recent trials (MRC CLL3 and LRF CLL4) have only randomised patients with Binet stages B, C and A progressive. When survival is considered in those two trials by stage, the value of this clinical parameter is not apparent (Figures 12.2 and 12.3) as stage A progressive patients (defined by short lymphocyte doubling time, downward trend in Hb and/or platelet count and increasing organomegaly) fare similarly to those with stage B. The analysis of outcome by prognostic factors in the MRC CLL3 trial, which entered 418 patients, showed in the multivariate analysis that the main factors were performance status ($p = 0.0001$), percentage of blood lymphocytes ($p = 0.001$), sex ($p = 0.007$) and age ($p = 0.009$), but not stage.

All the UK CLL trials, including CLL4 (Figure 12.4), have shown a significant survival advantage for females over males. Although there is a higher proportion of women with stage A and more men have stages B and C, the better prognosis of

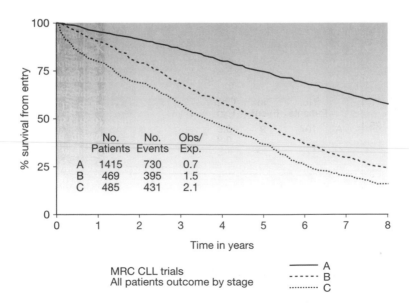

Figure 12.1 MRC CLL trials: All patients – outcome by stage.

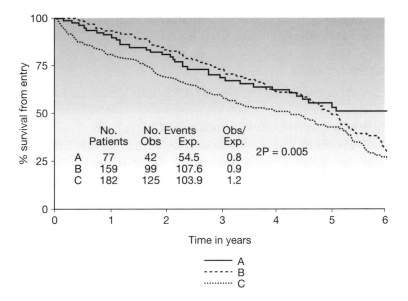

Figure 12.2 MRC CLL trials (October 1999): outcome by Binet stage.

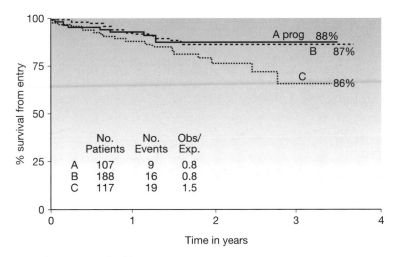

Figure 12.3 CLL4 – survival by stage.

women is independent of stage, age and response to therapy. Furthermore, even though age is an unfavourable prognostic feature and women with CLL tend to be older than men, they still fare better. Possible explanations for the better survival of females include their better response to treatment and the lower proportion of poor responders compared with males. One additional factor that may contribute to their better outcome is that at least twice as many females have mutated immunoglobulin genes VH genes compared with males.

Despite the better prognosis for good responders to treatment (Figures 12.5 and 12.6), large randomised trials (Rai *et al.* 2000; Leporrier *et al.* 2001) have failed to show a survival advantage for those randomised to fludarabine, despite achieving higher response rates. The issue in CLL is that responses to second-line therapies in non-responders to the first-line therapy improve survival and, therefore, even out prognosis. This was seen in the MRC CLL3NR study for non-responders to chlorambucil with or without epirubicin, who experienced excellent responses to fludarabine (Table 12.1). The importance of crossover therapy in CLL was apparent in the Cancer and Leukemia Group B (CALGB) trial (Rai *et al.* 2000), where 40% of non-responders achieved a good response to fludarabine, but only 7% of non-responders to fludarabine responded after crossing over to chlorambucil.

One of the groups in which prognosis and probability of disease progression seems important to be predicted beforehand is stage A CLL. The MRC CLL3A observational study collected diagnostic data on 551 patients. From the analysis of prognostic factors, both the lymphocyte doubling time (poor prognosis when less than 12 months) and the French sub-staging (A' vs A"; worse for A": Hb <12 and/or lymphocytes >30) were shown to be the most important and statistically significant independent prognostic factors ($2p < 0.001$). These observations are very relevant and need to be considered when current proposals for new therapeutic trials for stage A

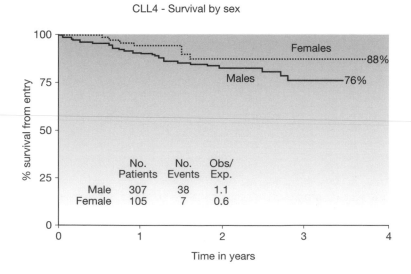

Figure 12.4 CLL4 – survival by sex.

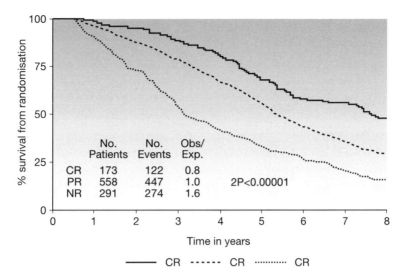

Figure 12.5 MRC CLL Trials: All patients – outcome by response.

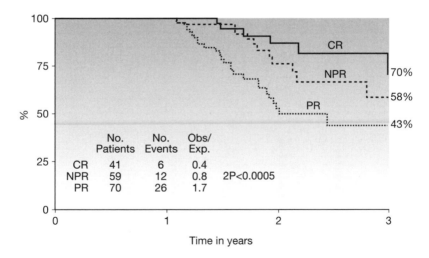

Figure 12.6 CLL4 – progression free survival by response. Landmark analysis from one year.

are planned with treatment modalities based on biological parameters of the disease such as VH mutations, CD38 expression, etc.

The current CLL4 trial has a comprehensive range of laboratory studies with new biological and laboratory parameters that will help confirm the prognostic value of

Table 12.1 Responses to fludarabine in primary non-responders to Chl or Chl+Epi

Response	No of patients* (%)
CR	13 (17)
PR	50 (64)
NR	15 (19)

VH mutations, expression of CD38 and ZAP70, and features detected by fluorescent *in situ* hybridisation (FISH) such as 11q, 6q, 17p (p53) deletions and trisomy 12. Of particular importance will be the behaviour of patients according to these parameters to the new treatment modalities tested, such as the response to purine analogues. CLL4 does not collect data on stable stage A patients; thus the above analysis of CLL3A will be important for any future study on stage A patients.

MRC CLL3 trial

This CLL trial ran from 1990 to 1997 and randomised 418 patients. It compared chlorambucil (given at 10 mg/m^2 × 6 days) with a combination of chlorambucil plus epirubicin (50 mg/m^2 on day 1), both treatments repeated at 4-weekly intervals. With a median follow-up of 5 years there was no survival difference between the two regimens (Catovsky *et al.* 2000). Responses are summarised in Table 12.2 for 350 patients with information after 1 year of treatment when the maximum responses were recorded. When responses with chlorambucil or the combination were assessed at 6 months, the rate of complete response (CR) was lower (9% chlorambucil, 18% chlorambucil plus epirubicin). There were no major differences in toxicity except for more thrombocytopenia with chlorambucil ($p = 0.03$) but less neutropenia ($p = 0.08$). The combination produced significantly more nausea, alopecia and mucositis.

Table 12.2 Response by treatment allocation

	Chl	Chl+Epi
CR	19%	22%
PR	58%	59%
NR	23%	19%
No pts	171	179

The information on CLL3 was incorporated in the overview of the CLL Trialists' Collaborative Group (1999), which showed no survival advantage for combinations with anthracyclines, including cyclophosphamide, doxorubicin, vincristine, and prednisone (CHOP). The issue of chlorambucil dose needs a comment here. As shown in Table 12.3, the dose of chlorambucil used is different in various trials and appears to influence response rates. The complete responses in the CALGB trial (Rai *et al.* 2000) and the German CLL5 trial are in single figures and lower than when higher doses are used, particularly the most intensive regimen used by Jaksic *et al.* (1997) Therefore, when chlorambucil was proposed as control arm in CLL4, the dose suggested was 70 mg/m², and this is currently in use.

Table 12.3 The dose of chlorambucil may influence response rates

Trial	Monthly dose	CR rate
CALGB trial	40mg/m²	3%
CLL5 – (German)	40mg/m²	7%
CLL3 – (MRC)	60mg/m²	19%
CLL4 – (LRF)	70mg/m²	
Robak *et al.* 2000	84mg/m²*	12%
Jaksic *et al.* 1997	150–180mg/m²	59%

* With prednisolone 30mg/m² × 7 days.

LRF CLL4

CLL4 is the most comprehensive trial thus far and incorporates several important elements in addition to establishing the possible benefits of the purine analogue fludarabine used alone or in combination with cyclophosphamide (FC) as first-line treatment for patients with Binet stages B, C and A progressive. Half of the patients received chlorambucil and the other half either fludarabine or FC. There is central review of diagnosis based on markers (immunophenotype) and morphology, quality of life assessment through a questionnaire sent regularly to patients, extensive laboratory investigations to examine new prognostic factors such as deletions at 6q, 11q, 13q, 17p and trisomy 12 tested by FISH, expression of CD38 and ZAP 70 examined by triple colour flow cytometry as surrogates for IgVH mutations and actual VH mutations by PCR analysis. Finally, randomised evaluation of the DiSC assay (Bosanquet *et al.* 1999) to test *in vitro* drug sensitivity for non-responders or early relapsers.

The treatment rationale and main features of CLL4 are summarised in Tables 12.4 and 12.5. The trial started in February 1999 with the intravenous formulation of fludarabine and cyclophosphamide but since February 2001 it has incorporated the oral formulation, which has equal efficacy and greater convenience. It might be possible and, indeed, of interest as a by-product of CLL4 to examine the relative efficacy of both administration routes, a question that has never been addressed specifically in a randomised trial.

Table 12.4 Rationale for CLL4

* Fludara high CR rates as first line (Keating *et al.* 1998)
* Synergistic potential of fludarabine + cyclophosphamide (O'Brien *et al.* 2001)
* Responders in CLL do better than non-responders (Tables 12.5 and 12.6)

Table 12.5 Features for CLL4

- First line fludarabine
- Combination of fludarabine plus cyclophosphamide
- Bone marrow biopsy to assess response
- Randomised evaluation of the DiSC assay for non-responders and relapses (Bosanquet *et al.* 1999)

The higher complete response rates reported by the M. D. Anderson Cancer Center (Houston, Texas) group with FC (O'Brien *et al.* 2001) have been confirmed by a phase II study of the German CLL group (Hallek *et al.* 2001). LRF CLL4 is one of the few clinical trials worldwide that is looking prospectively at FC in a phase III randomised fashion.

CLL4, in addition to covering all aspects of CLL – diagnosis, treatment and prognosis – is thus far the most successful CLL trial in the UK, and 10% of the participants are from centres in other countries (Argentina, Russia, Italy, New Zealand, Greece, etc.). The original target of 500 randomised patients has been reached in fewer than 5 years (latest recruitment figures are 697 by 28 June 2004). A new target of 750 has now been agreed, to increase the statistical power to 80% to detect a 10% difference in survival from 40% to 50% (from 65% power with 500 patients). This means a likelihood of closing recruitment early in 2005 if current rates of randomisation continue. Neither of the two large randomised trials using fludarabine as first line were published at the time CLL4 started. The CALGB study (Rai *et al.* 2000) randomised 544 patients, and the French Cooperative Group (Leporrier *et al.* 2001) 938 patients, but both included three treatment arms. Neither of them showed a significant survival difference for fludarabine, but neither was sufficiently large to detect or rule out a difference of 10%. The results of CLL4 could also enrich any meta-analysis of randomised trials using purine analogues as first line.

End points of CLL4 are summarised in Table 12.6; they do not include only survival as in past trials. A preliminary view of survival of CLL4, compared with its predecessors CLL trials 1, 2 and 3, shows encouraging signs that patients in CLL4 are doing better (Figure 12.7) and this is not just due to the new treatments but also to better results with chlorambucil which (as discussed above) is used with a more intensive schedule.

Table 12.6 End points of CLL4

- Overall response rate
- Survival
- Progression free survival
- Time to progression
- Toxicity
- Quality of life

CLL4 uses (as did CLL3) the Binet *et al.* (1981) staging system. Assessment of response is very similar, although not identical, to the criteria published by the National Cancer Institute of the USA (Cheson *et al.* 1996). As CLL4 is still ongoing, details of results of the various modalities are not available. Toxicity is, however, closely monitored. Toxicity data on the first 304 patients are summarised in Tables 12.7–12.9. Of note is the greater degree of neutropenia with the combination of fludarabine and cyclophosphamide (Table 12.7) and slightly more episodes of infection (Table 12.8). Participants have been advised on greater vigilance of blood counts in patients receiving the combination, particularly after the first few courses, and to readily prescribe growth factors, e.g. G-CSF, to prevent neutropenic sepsis, episodes of which have already been observed and duly reported as serious adverse events (SAEs). Other toxicities (Table 12.9) also reflect the greater intensity of the FC combination. Diarrhoea is seen at the end of the 5-day oral courses of fludarabine, but this is easily controlled and is of no major clinical consequence.

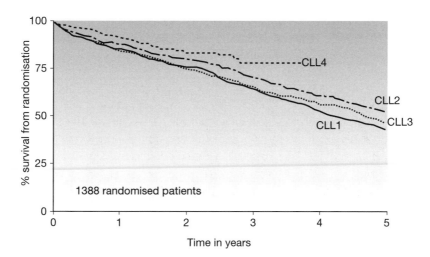

Figure 12.7 MRC CLL trials.

Table 12.7 CLL4 – Haematological toxicity (based on 304 pts)

	Chl	Fludarabine	Fludarabine + cyclophosphamide
Neutropenia (<1 × 10⁹/l)	32%	42%	53%
Thrombocytop. (<50 × 10⁹/l)	14%	12%	6%

Table 12.8 CLL4 – infections (based on 304 pts)

Days in hospital	Chlorambucil	Fludarabine	Fludarabine + cyclophosphamide
<4 weeks	23%	36%	31%
≥4 weeks	1%	5%	9%
Febrile episodes (>1)	30%	29%	36%

Table 12.9 CLL4 – GI and other toxicities (grades 1–3) (based on 304 pts)

	Chlorambucil	Fludarabine	Fludarabine + cyclophosphamide
Nausea/vomiting	42%	30%	51%
Alopecia	8%	10%	23%
Mucositis	12%	18%	7%
Diarrhoea	19%	25%	12%

CLL4 is a model trial which reflects the advances in the management of CLL and greater knowledge of its biology at molecular level. The results of laboratory studies, assessment of treatment responses and identification of prognostic categories will bring CLL to the level already achieved in the acute leukaemias, both acute lymphocytic leukemia (ALL) and acute myeloid leukemia (AML), and allow tailoring of therapy according to prognostic categories.

Our personal experience with the DiSC assay (assessment of *in vitro* sensitivity of CLL cells to drugs) shows that high doses of methylprednisolone can overcome the well-known drug resistance of CLL with acquired p53 abnormalities (Thornton *et al.* 2003). A similar effect has been suggested with the monoclonal antibody alemtuzumab (Campath-1H), a new very effective agent (Keating *et al.* 2002; Stilgenbauer and Dohner, 2002), along with rituximab for future trials in resistant/relapsed patients. Indeed, some of these modalities may be incorporated in the next generation of CLL trials at an early stage of the treatment protocols. The better survival and response to treatment of women remains an interesting observation which may translate into clinical benefits if the reasons for this more favourable prognosis can be established.

References

Binet, J. L., Catovsky, D., Chandra, P., Dighiero, G., Montserrat, E., Rai, K. R. & Sawitsky, A. (1981). Proposal for a revised prognostic staging system, Report from the international workshop on CLL. *British Journal of Haematology* **98**, 365–367.

Bosanquet, A. G., Johnson, S. A. & Richards, S. M. (1999). Prognosis for fludarabine therapy of chronic lymphocytic leukaemia based on ex vivo drug response by DiSC assay. *British Journal of Haematology* **106**, 71–77.

Catovsky, D., Hamblin, T. J. & Richards, S. (2000). UK Medical Research Council CLL3–A randomised trial of the addition of epirubicin to standard chlorambucil treatment. *Blood* **96**, 754a (abstract 3263).

Catovsky, D., Richards, S., Fooks, J. & Hamblin, T. J. (1991). CLL trials in the United Kingdom. *Leukemia & Lymphoma* (Suppl.), 105–111.

Catovsky, D., Fooks, J. & Richards, S. (1989). Prognostic factors in chronic lymphocytic leukaemia: the importance of age, sex and response to treatment in survival. A report from the MRC CLL 1 trial. MRC Working Party on Leukaemia in Adults. *British Journal of Haematology* **72**, 141–149.

Cheson, B. D., Bennett, J. M., Grever, M., Kay, N., Keating, M. J., O'Brien, S., Rai, K. R. (1996). National Cancer Institute-sponsored Working Group guidelines for chronic lymphocytic leukemia: revised guidelines for diagnosis and treatment. *Blood* **87**, 4990–4997.

CLL Trialists' Collaborative Group (1999). Chemotherapeutic options in chronic lymphocytic leukemia: A meta-analysis of the randomised trials. *Journal of the National Cancer Institute* **91**, 861–868.

Hallek, M., Schmitt, B., Wilheim, M., Busch, R., Krober, A., Fostitsch, H.P., Sezer, O., Herold, M., Knauf, W., Wendtner, C.M., Kuse, R., Freund, M., Franke, A., Schriever, F., Nerl, C., Dohner, H., Thiel, E., Hiddemann, W., Brittinger, G. & Emmerich, B. (2001). Fludarabine plus cyclophosphamide is an efficient treatment for advanced chronic lymphocytic leukaemia (CLL): results of a phase II study of the German CLL study group. *British Journal of Haematology* **114**, 342–348.

Jaksic, B., Brugiatelli, M., Krc, I., Losonczi, H., Holowiecki, J., Planinc-Peraica, A., Kusec, R., Morabito, F., Iacopino, P. & Lutz, D. (1997). High dose chlorambucil versus Binet's modified cyclophosphamide, doxorubicin, vincristine and prednisone regimen in the treatment of patients with advanced B-cell chronic lymphocytic leukaemia. Result of an international multicenter randomized trial. *Cancer* **79**, 2107–2114.

Keating, M.J., O'Brien, S., Lerner, S., Koller, C., Beran, M., Robertson, L.E., Freireich, E.J., Estey, E. & Kantarjian, H. (1998). Long-term follow up of patients with chronic lymphocytic leukaemia (CLL) receiving fludarabine regimens as initial therapy. *Blood* **92**, 1165–1171.

Keating, M. J., Flinn, I., Jain, V., Binet, J. L., Hillmen, P., Byrd, J., Albitar, M., Brettman, L., Santabarbara, P., Wacker, B., Rai, K. R. (2002). Therapeutic role of alemtuzumab (Campath-1H) in patients who have failed fludarabine: results of a large international study. *Blood* **99**, 3554–3561.

Leporrier, M., Chevret, S., Cazin, B., Boudjerra, N., Feugier, P., Desablens, B., Rapp, M. J., Jaubert, J., Autrand, C., Divine, M., Dreyfus, B., Maloum, K., Travade, P., Dighiero, G., Binet, J. L. & Chastang, C.; French Cooperative Group on Chronic Lymphocytic Leukemia (2001). Ransomized comparison of fludarabine, CAP, and CHOP in 938 previously untreated stage B and C chronic lymphocytic leukemia patients. *Blood* **98**, 2319–2325.

O'Brien, S. M., Kantarjian, H. M., Cortes, J., Beran, M., Koller, C. A., Giles, F. J., Lerner, S., Keating, M. (2001). Results of the fludarabine and cyclophosphamide combination regimen in chronic lymphocytic leukemia. *Journal of Clinical Oncology* **19**, 1414–1420.

Rai, K. R., Peterson, B. L., Applebaum, F. R., Kolitz, J., Elias, L., Shepherd, L., Hines, J., Threatte, G. A., Larson, R. A., Cheson, B. D. & Schiffer, C.A. (2000). Fludarabine compared with chlorambucil as primary therapy for chronic lymphocytic leukemia. *New England Journal of Medicine* **343**, 1750–1757.

Robak, T., Blonski, J. Z., Kasznicki, M., Blasinska-Morawiec, M., Krykowski, E., Dmoszynska, A., Mrugala-Spiewak, H., Skotnicki, A. B., Nowak, W., Konopka, L.,

Ceglarek, B., Maj, S., Dwilewicz-Trojaczek, J., Hellmann, A., Urasinski, I., Zdziarska, B., Kotlarek-Haus, S., Potoczek, S. & Grieb, P. (2000). Cladribine with prednisone versus chlorambucil with prednisone as first-line therapy in chronic lymphocytic leukemia: report of a prospective, randomized, multicenter trial. *Blood* **96**, 2723–2729.

Stilgenbauer, S. & Dohner, H. (2002). Campath-1H-induced complete remission of chronic lymphocytic leukemia despite p53 gene mutation and resistance to chemotherapy. *New England Journal of Medicine* **347**, 452–453.

Thornton, P. D., Matutes, E., Bosanquet, A. G., Lakhani, A. K., Grech, H., Ropner, J. E., Joshi, R., Mackie, P. H., Douglas, I. D., Bowcock, S. J. & Catovsky, D. (2003). High dose methylprednisolone can induce remissions in CLL patients with p53 abnormalities. *Annals of Hematology* **82**, 759–765.

Chapter 13

Clinical practice guidelines for the management of chronic lymphocytic leukaemia

David G. Oscier and Stephen A. Johnson

Introduction

The production of guidelines designed to aid clinicians in applying the criteria for diagnosis, and establishing the standards of treatment for the management of specific diseases, is currently seen to be the responsibility of specialist professional groups. Guidelines for use in the United Kingdom covering haematological disorders are generally provided by the British Society of Haematology (BSH) through their professional standards committee, and the British Committee for Standards in Haematology (BCSH), which has task forces leading the process for general haematology, haemostasis and thrombosis, blood transfusion and haemato-oncology. The guidelines for the management of chronic lymphocytic leukaemia (CLL) were commissioned by the Haemato-Oncology task force of BCSH from the UK CLL forum, a group specialising in the management of CLL; this organisation became responsible for forming the writing committee, and preparing the document for approval and subsequent dissemination.

The process of producing guidelines must be rigorously controlled so that, as far as possible, the end result is an accurate and reliable document containing sound advice to the clinicians who will consult it for guidance. Although it is doubtful if the organisation responsible for the guidelines (in this case, the BSH), can be held legally responsible for their content, the advice they contain may be used in a wider context than solely for clinical management; the guideline text may, for instance, be used to define the distribution of service provision by hospitals, establish the ability of specialists to practise, or promote the interests of a manufacturing company in relation to a specific product.

Methods

The process of producing the CLL Guidelines is summarised in Figure 13.1. The early stages have already been outlined and consist of the commissioning process after which a writing group is formed. The convenor of this group selects experts in the field who will be responsible for production of the majority of the text. In addition he will invite a patient/lay member to ensure that the text is clearly written, and to

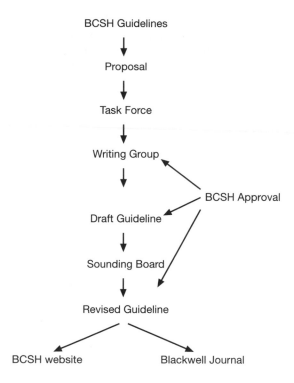

Figure 13.1 Production of BCSH Guidelines.

contribute to those areas which reflect the patient's perspective, such as communication of diagnosis and/or prognosis, and recommendation of external sources of information such as support groups or internet resources.

Guidance for the working group is offered by the BCSH to try to ensure that guidelines are produced to a uniform (high) standard and cover the necessity to declare any external source of funding or conflict of interest among the authors. The BCSH also recommends the incorporation of a disclaimer to emphasise the limited liability inherent in the guideline process. The current disclaimer reads as follows:

> *'While the advice and information contained in this guideline are believed to be true and accurate at the time of going to press, neither the authors nor the publishers can accept legal responsibility or liability for any errors or omissions that may be made.'*

At an early stage in the process of guideline production the working group need to plan the acquisition of the information required. An explicit strategy for the literature search must be defined and the source of pharmaco-economic risk benefit analyses should be identified. The overall rigor of the process of writing the guidelines, and the validity of the final document, is measured by use of the AGREE appraisal instrument (the AGREE Collaboration 2001), which provides a template for scoring all aspects of guideline production (Figure 13.2).

- Scope and purpose
- Stakeholder involvement
- Rigour of development
- Clarity and presentation
- Applicability
- Editorial independence

Figure 13.2 AGREE appraisal instrument.

An assessment of the strength of published evidence is required to clarify the reliability of cited literature, and the most commonly applied system for classification of evidence and grading of recommendations is that devised by the US Agency for Health Care Policy and Research (Figure 13.3). The guideline is designed to discuss the relevant evidence, provide clear conclusions, suggest standards that could be used as topics for audit, and state the intended review date of its advice.

Results

The UK CLL Forum guidelines working group consisted of eight individuals of whom six were haematologists (including two members of the BCSH Haemato-Oncology Task Force), one clinical oncologist and one patient representative. No external funding was used and no conflicts of interest likely to affect the contribution of individual authors were declared. The literature review involved the use of Medline and Pubmed searches under the heading 'chronic lymphocytic leukaemia' up to October 2003, and data presented at the American Society of Hematology and at the 10th International Workshop on CLL in 2003. The results of meta-analyses and phase 3 studies that had been published in abstract form were included. The guideline was laid out according to the standard BCSH format: summary, objectives, methods, recommendations.

Specific sections of the guideline covered the following topics: diagnosis, prognostic factors, indications for referral, communicating with patients, indications for treatment, treatment options, management of complications.

In accordance with BCSH requirements for guideline approval, the first draft was then circulated to members of the UK CLL Forum and approximately 60 (volunteer) UK haematologists. Their feedback was used to modify the document and produce a second draft. At this stage the guideline was submitted to the BCSH and accepted after a series of minor revisions were agreed. The BSH has now approved publication

Classification of grades of recommendations

A Requires at least one randomised controlled trial as part of a body of
literature of overall good quality and consistency addressing specific
recommendation
(Evidence levels Ia Ib)

B Requires the availability of well conducted clinical studies but no
randomised clinical trials on the topic of recommendation
(Evidence levels IIa IIb III)

C Requires evidence obtained from expert commitee reports or opinions
and/or clinical experiences of respected authorities. Indicates an
absence of directly applicable clinical studies of good quality
(Evidence Level IV)

Classification of evidence levels

Ia Evidence obtained from meta-anlysis of randomised controlled trials.

Ib Evidence obtained from at least one randomised controlled trial.

IIa Evidence obtained from at least one well-designed study without
randomisation.

IIb Evidence obtained from at least one other type of well-designed equal
experimental study.

III Evidence obtained from well-designed non-experimental descriptive
studies, correlation studies and case studies.

IV Evidence obtained from expert committee reports or opinions and/or
clinical experiences of respected authorities.

Figure 13.3 Criteria for levels of evidence and grades of recommendation.

of the guideline on the BCSH website (www.bcshguidelines.com) where it can be
consulted without restriction. Despite the extensive review process already
undertaken, it is the policy of the BCSH to promote publication of its guidelines in a
peer-reviewed journal. The CLL guidelines were submitted to the *British Journal of
Haematology*, and after the editorial process, which included review by two
independent non-UK referees (usually a haematologist and a guideline expert), a
modified guideline has been published (Oscier *et al.* 2004).

Discussion

The production and promulgation of guidelines may have substantial benefits for
clinicians, giving them access to evidence-based advice concerning the intentions of

proven benefit, and discouraging the use of ineffective treatments. An up-to-date and rigorously produced guideline also has a clear educational function, and in addition may form the basis for audit of clinical management. It may also identify areas of care for which greater resources are required. There are, however, potential limitations associated with guideline use, especially if recommendations are incorrect or outdated. The sponsoring organisation has an obligation to ensure that its guidelines are produced to rigorous standards even if strict legal liability is denied. Other shortcomings of the wholesale application of guidelines are that they are often too simplistic for the problems of individual patients, and if they are uncritically applied will result in the erosion of clinical judgement. As a safeguard against the possibility of the guideline incorporating clinically inappropriate advice, it is important that the major input into the text, and the production of treatment algorithms should be from a working group with a majority of practising clinicians.

Reference

The AGREE Collaboration (2001). Appraisal of Guidelines for Research and Evaluation (AGREE) Instrument. www.agreecollaboration.org

Oscier, D., Fegan, C., Hillmen, P., Illidge, T., Johnson, S., Maguire, P., Matutes, E. & Milligan, D.; Guidelines Working Group of the UK CLL Forum. British Committee for Standards in Haematology (2004). Guidelines on the diagnosis and management of chronic lymphocytic leukaemia. *British Journal of Haematology* **125**, 294–317.

Index

17-AAG (geldanamycin) 128, 130
aciclovir, prophylactic use in
    alemtuzumab therapy 147, 148
acquired angio-oedema (AAE) 160,
    162
  treatment 168
activation-induced cytidine deaminase
    (AID) 40–41
adenoviral infection, association with
    alemtuzumab therapy 147
adhesion receptors 51–52
age, prognostic significance 180, 181
age at diagnosis in familial CLL 4
AGREE appraisal instrument 193
alemtuzumab (Campath-IH) xi, xii,
    xvi, 94, 116, 134, 135, 188
  anti-viral prophylaxis 148
  in early disease 86
  immunosuppressive effect 147
  response rates 106
  second-line use 104
  use in stem-cell transplantation 119
  value in p53 abnormalities 29
alkylating agents xi, 89, 91, 99
  in second-line therapy 100–101
  see also chlorambucil
allogeneic stem cell transplantation
    xii, xiii, 95, 113, 117–18
  low-intensity 118–119
  unrelated donors 119
alopecia as complication of treatment
    xvi
$\alpha_4\beta_1$ expression 51
androgens, use in acquired angio-
    oedema 168
angio-oedema, acquired xv, 160, 162
  treatment 168
ankylosing spondylitis 159
anti-B-cell antibodies, use in purging
    116
antibiotic prophylaxis xiv–xv, 148
antiCD20 antibody *see* rituximab
antiCD52 antibody *see* alemtuzumab
    (Campath-IH)

anticipation in CLL 4
antigens, role in CLL development 45,
    46–48
anti-neutrophil cytoplasmic antibodies
    160
antisense oligonucleotides (ASOs) xiv,
    133–134
anti-viral prophylaxis 148
apicidin 132
apoptosis
  effect of bortezomib (PS-341) 129
  effect of FR901228 (depsipeptide)
    131
  effect of triterpenoids 130
  role in CLL 125, 126
  role of P2X7 receptor 10
apoptosis induction 135–136
association studies 7
ataxia telangiectasia mutated (ATM)
    gene 8–9, 23, 24, 27, 43
  prognostic significance 82
atypical CLL x
  cell morphology 66, 67, 68
autocrine cytokines 52–53
autoimmune disease xv, 48, 53, 54,
    157, 158
  autoantibody secretion by CLL cells
    161–162
  immune thrombocytopenia (ITP) 158
  neutropenia 159
  non-haematological 159–161
  pure red-cell aplasia (PRCA) 159
  T-cell hypothesis 164
  treatment 164–168
  triggered by treatment 162–164
autoimmune haemolytic anaemia
    (AIHA) xv, 157–158, 162
  treatment 164–166, 167
  treatment-triggered 162–163
autologous stem cell transplantation
    xii, xiii, 95, 113–114
  conditioning regimens 117
  effect on quality of life 117
  patient selection bias in clinical
    studies 115
  purging 116
  stem-cell mobilisation 115